Dr. Sebi Coo[illegible]

200+ Mouth Watering Recipes to Drastically Improve Your Health, Cleanse Your Liver and Detox the Body through the Alkaline Diet

Neal Graham

Table of Contents

Introduction

Dr. Sebi felt the Western solution to illness was unsuccessful. He held that acidity and mucus — for starters, bacteria, and viruses — induced sickness.

A big dietary hypothesis is that illness can exist only in acidic conditions. To avoid or eliminate the disease, the purpose of the diet is to maintain alkaline conditions in the body. The official website of the food offers botanical medicines helping to detoxify the body.

Methodology

Often, stretching for the additional mile, you get to the areas you had only dreamed about. They were going well on Dr. Sebi's alkaline diet, which will be the battle that ultimately contributes to a balanced lifestyle. Dr. Sebi's alkaline diet is an assumption that certain products, such as berries, vegetables, roots, and legumes, leave a chemical residue or ash behind in the body. The body is strengthened by the critical ingredients of rock, such as calcium, magnesium, titanium, zinc, and copper. The avoidance of asthma, malnutrition, exhaustion, and even cancer is an alkaline diet. Here are ten strategies to adopt this diet effectively, following these strategies to see results immediately:

1. **Drink water.** Water is probably our body's most famous (after oxygen) resource. Drink between 8-10 glasses of water to keep the body well hydrated (filtered to cleaned).
2. **Avoid acidic drinks like tea, coffee, or soda.** Our body also attempts to regulate acid and alkaline content. There is no need to blink in carbonated beverages as the body refuses carbon dioxide as waste!
3. **Breathe.** Oxygen is the explanation that our body works, and if you provide the body with adequate oxygen, it should perform better. Sit back and enjoy two to five minutes of slow breaths. Nothing is easier than performing Yoga.
4. **Avoid food with preservatives and food colours.** Our body has not been programmed to absorb such substances, and the body then absorbs them or retains them as fat, so they do not damage the liver. Chemicals create acids, such that the body neutralizes them either by generating cholesterols or blanching iron from the RBCs (leading to anaemia) or by extracting calcium from bones (osteoporosis).
5. **Avoid artificial sweeteners.** These sweeteners, which tend to be high in low fat, are potentially detrimental to the body. In addition, Saccharin, a primary ingredient in sweeteners, triggers cancer. Keep away from these things, therefore. Go for less healthy food, still a decent one.
6. **Exercise.** Alkaline and the acidic element will also be matched. A little acid (because of muscles) often regulates natural bodywork.

7. **Satiate your urges for a snack by eating vegetables or soaked nuts.** Whenever we are thirsty, we still consume a little fast food. Establish a tradition of consuming fresh vegetables or almonds, even walnuts.

Chapter 1: Doctor Sebi's Food List

Many individuals in the U.S. suffer from different diseases ranging from cancer, hypertension, diabetes, mental disabilities, and many more. Many of these junks and fast foods are disease-causing substances (contains too much acid) not because they contain pathogens but because they contain elements such as an increasing amount of acid that increase weight and clogged up in the body.

The accumulation of all these substances in the body brings about an increased amount of fatty acids and cholesterol, which later blocks up the blood vessels and hinders the free flow of blood.

Many of these substances cause genetic materials in the body to make a mistake and bring about the growth of abnormal cells, which subsequently result in cancer.

Nowadays, dieters have embraced the intake of alkaline food not only because they know the importance of clean and prolong life.

Acidic foods are majorly the foods we eat. Such foods are meat, grains, eggs, fish, alcohol, etc. These foods increase the body's acidic level. The intake of alkaline foods will cause your blood to become soluble and therefore inhibit you from having diseases.

When you take a plant diet that has a reduced acid diet, it replaces the animal protein with excess acid. This will promote your kidney because it makes it reduce its work of removing the excess acids present in animal diets.

Besides, bone diseases and many bones associated problems are at times are related to the consumption of some foods that are high in acid. Then, to avoid any bone infections in the body, you must endeavour to eat alkaline diets.

The foods designed by Dr. Sebi are straightforward to acquire around you, and they are cheap and do expensive activities in your body. These foods make you remain lean, clean, and healthy.

Dr. Sebi classified the foods into different categories. These categories are:

- Fruits
- Vegetables
- Alkaline Grains
- Alkaline Sugars

Vegetables

- Cucumber
- Tomatillo
- Turnip greens.
- Wakame
- Onions
- Dandelion greens
- Cherry and plum tomato
- Dulse
- Garbanzo beans
- Izote flower and leaf
- Kale
- Mushrooms except for Shitake
- Arame
- Wild Arugula
- Avocado
- Amaranth
- Bell Pepper
- Chayote
- Hijiki
- Nopales
- Nori
- Zucchini
- Watercress
- Lettuce except for iceberg
- Olives
- Purslane verdolaga
- Squash
- Okra

Fruits

- Apples
- Pears
- Limes
- Mango
- Berries
- Melons
- Prickly pear
- Cherries
- Soursops
- Dates
- Figs
- Grapes
- Prunes
- Raisins
- Papayas
- Bananas
- Cantaloupe
- Currants
- Orange
- Soft jelly coconuts
- Peaches
- Plums

Alkaline Grains

- Spelt
- Fonio
- Quinoa
- Rye
- Kamut
- Tef
- Wild rice
- Amaranth

Alkaline Sugars

- 100% Pure agave syrup extracted from cactus
- Dried date sugar

Diets Designed by Dr. Sebi

The diets designed by Dr. Sebi are essential for the prevention and cure of cancer disease and many other conditions. All sufferers of cancer disease are expected to consume only foods approved by Dr. Sebi, although the diets might be severe for those who are addicted to acidic foods such as rice, soy, beans, alcohol, junks, and many more.

List of Foods to Avoid in Dr. Sebi's Diet

Some foods are disregarded in Dr. Sebi's food list because you must do away with them. Most of these foods could be dangerous for your health, especially for cancer patients.

These foods contain an increasing amount of acidic contents and are not advised to be taken by a cancer patient. Although these foods are suitable for the mouth, they are not good for the body. Dr. Sebi tagged them as forbidden foods. These foods are listed below:

- Alcoholic beverages
- Fish and seafood
- Meat of all kind
- Poultry products
- Colorants and flavours
- Processed foods
- Canned foods and fruits
- Soy and soy products
- Corn
- Genetically modified organism fruits
- Eggs
- Wheat
- Seedless fruits
- Foods with yeast or other components such as baking powder
- Fast foods
- Sugar
- Foods fortified with vitamins and minerals
- Garlic
- Genetically modified organism vegetables
- Dairy foods

Approved Products

While food plays the most significant part in the Dr. Sebi diet, there are products that he recommends you take. Various sites sell Dr. Sebi supplements. Some are more luxurious and expensive than others, but they are all the same things. The goal of the supplements is to provide your body with nutrients that it needs to function correctly. Some supplements are specific to men and women as well, so make sure that you pay attention. Most websites will also provide you with grouped products that offer you everything you need for general health or to heal a specific ailment.

Iron Plus

Iron plus is meant to help purify the entire body. It contains chaparral, which, as we have talked about, is a powerful antioxidant. Iron plus also contains:

- Bugleweed
- Palo guaco
- Hombre grande
- Blue vervain
- Chaparral
- Elderberry

Green Food

This is a multi-mineral supplement that is made up of herbs from Africa and offers chlorophyll-rich food that nourished the body. It contains ortiga, which is well known as an anti-inflammatory. It can also help with gout, rheumatism, influenza, hemorrhage, cardiovascular system, locomotor system disorders, gastrointestinal tract disorders, urinary tract infections, and kidney disorders. It is also great at helping poor circulation and purifying the blood. Ortiga has also been used to improve the symptoms of hay fever. Green food contains:

- Bladderwrack
- Nopal
- Tila
- Nettle

Bromide Plus Powder/Bromide Plus Capsules

This is meant to help your thyroid gland and bones. It is excellent for people who suffer from dysentery, respiratory issues, pulmonary illnesses, and bad breath. It is a natural diuretic, improves the digestive system, regulates the bowels, and suppresses the appetite. It contains bladderwrack, which is a seaweed that lives in the Baltic Sea, Atlantic Ocean, and the Pacific Ocean. It is one of the sources of iodine. It is full of mannitol, alginic, potassium, bromine, and beta-carotene. It contains bladderwrack and Irish sea moss.

Bio Ferro Tonic/Bio Ferro Capsules

Bio Ferro contains the right ingredients to purify and nourish the blood. It includes a yellow dock root, which is an herb that acts as a digestive bitter to help improve digestion. It is a detoxifier and blood purifier and especially helps the liver. Yellow dock root also helps the metabolism of fats and stimulates bile production. It can also help with bowel movements and get rid of waste lingering in the intestinal tract. It will also increase urination. Bio Ferro contains:

- Cocolmeca
- Yellow dock root
- Burdock root
- Chaparral
- Elderberry

Bio ferro capsules work the same way as the tonic. They have slightly different ingredients even though they do the same thing. The capsules contain:

- Yellow dock root
- Nopal
- Nettle
- Burdock root
- Chaparral

Banju

The banju tonic is made from potent ingredients to make a tonic that helps to stimulate the central nervous system and brain. It contains:

- Bugleweed
- Valerian root
- Burdock root
- Blue vervain
- Elderberry

Body Care

1. Uterine Oil and Wash

As you can presumption by the name, this is meant for women. This helps to cleanse and restore the flora and fauna of the vagina. The red clover in the wash acts as a blood purifier, improves circulation, and acts as an expectorant. It also contains isoflavones and flavonoids, which help to produce estrogen. Red clover is excellent at treating conditions that are associated with menopause. The ingredients in the wash include:

- Red clover
- Sage
- Arnica

- Lupulo

2. Tooth Powder

This is a natural powder that you can use as a toothpaste that will help stop gum disease and tooth decay. It contains Encino and myrrh gum powder.

3. Hair Food Oil

This is meant to nourish the scalp and hair. It is gentle on the skin so that it can be used every day. It helps stimulate hair growth. It contains:

- French vanilla
- Coconut oil
- Batana oil
- Olive oil

4. Eyewash

This product naturally cleanses and nourishes the eye. It contains the only eyebright, which is commonly used to help treat many different eye diseases. It can also aid to reduce the inflammation in the eye caused by conjunctivitis and blepharitis.

5. Eva Salve

This salve is meant to tone and nourish the skin. The unique combination of ingredients in eva salve provides natural minerals the skin needs like potassium phosphate, fluorine, and calcium, which your skin needs to maintain elasticity. It also contains sage which is a powerful antioxidant that helps to fight off free radical damage. Eva salve contains:

- Manzo
- Eucalyptus
- Sage
- Arnica
- Olive oil
- Lily of the valley
- Nopal
- Shea butter
- Estro

Herbal Teas

- Stomach relief tea
- Stress relief tea
- Immune support tea
- Energy booster tea
- Cold and cough tea
- Blood pressure balance tea

Foods to Avoid

Any foods that are not covered in the Dr. Sebi vitamins manual aren't accredited, which includes:

- Canned fruit or vegetables
- Seedless fruit
- Eggs
- Dairy
- Fish
- Red meat
- Rooster
- Soy products
- Processed meals, including take-out or eating place meals
- Fortified ingredients
- Wheat
- Sugar (except date sugar and agave syrup)
- Alcohol
- Yeast or foods rose with yeast
- Meals made with baking powder

Furthermore, many greens, grains, nuts, and seeds are banned on the diet. Only foods indexed inside the guide can be eaten. The food regimen limits any food this is processed, animal-primarily based, or made with leavening.

Chapter 2: How to Follow the Diet

Rules to Follow

To follow Dr. Sebi's diet, you need to strictly adhere to his rules, which are present on his website. Here is a list of his guidelines below:

1. Do not eat or drink any product or ingredient not mentioned in the approved list for the diet. It is not recommended and should never be consumed when following the diet.
2. You have to drink almost one gallon (or more than three liters) of water every day. It is recommended to drink spring water.
3. You have to take Dr. Sebi's mixtures or products one hour before consuming your medications.
4. You can take any of Dr. Sebi's mixtures/products together without any worry.
5. You need to follow the nutritional guidelines stringently and punctually take Dr. Sebi's mixtures/products daily.
6. You are not allowed to consume any animal-based food or hybrid products.
7. You are not allowed to consume alcohol or any kind of dairy product.
8. You are not allowed to consume wheat, only natural growing grains as listed in the nutritional guide
9. The grains mentioned in the nutritional guide can be available in different forms, like pasta and bread, in different health food stores. You can consume them.
10. Do not use fruits from cans; also, seedless fruits are not recommended for consumption.
11. You are not allowed to use a microwave to reheat your meals.

How to Prepare the Body

It should be clear that it is a restrictive diet low in calories. Many people believe that because of this reason, it cannot be used as a standard way to lose weight as it puts too much stress on the body of a new dieter. Because it is low in calories and an intensive diet, weight loss can be seen, but the person needs to assess whether they are capable of handling a low caloric diet. Being too ambitious with this diet might turn fatal, so if you want to try the diet, be careful!

This diet has been suggested to be followed throughout one's entire life, which might not be possible for a new dieter. With any diet, if you start cutting foods strongly and then revert to your old routine of eating unhealthy meals, the chances are that the weight loss and benefits you see will get reversed. This is a risk in this diet as well. When starting, set reasonable goals and don't go too strongly. Let your body first get used to it and then start setting up more ambitious goals.

Meal Plan

Starting the diet can be daunting, so here is a list of meal ideas that you can copy from. For the first few days, follow it so that you get used to the diet.

Breakfast

1. Banana pancakes with agave syrup (more than one is recommended).

2. A strawberry and banana smoothie with added hemp seeds and water.

3. Cooked quinoa with coconut milk (pure) and agave syrup for sweetness (add a fruit of your choice as well).

Lunch

1. A salad made up of kale, tomatoes, onions, avocados, and chickpeas with olive oil and dressing of herbs.

2. A pizza made with spelt flour, Brazil nut cheese topped with different vegetables like tomatoes, etc.

3. A pasta made of spelt with different vegetables, and lime and olive oil dressings.

Evening Snack

1. A smoothie made by cucumbers, kale, a few pieces of ginger, and one or two apples.

2. Herbal tea accompanied by the fruit of your choice.

3. Blueberry muffins made by spelt and teff flour, coconut milk (pure), agave syrup, and blueberries.

Dinner

1. A wild rice stir-fry with vegetables of your choice.

2. A burger made up of spelt flour bread; tomatoes, onions, and kale as vegetables; and a chickpea patty.

3. Thick vegetable soup made up of zucchini, mushrooms, peppers, spices, sea salt, onions, and seaweed powder.

Drink Water

Smoothies are a drink, and by drinking them, you are ultimately fulfilling your water intake for the day. Dr. Sebi's diet requires you to drink one gallon of water daily, but that can be difficult. Dehydration is a serious problem that can lead to anxiety. To prevent that, you need to drink lots of water, which the smoothie diet helps you with.

What You Should Not Eat

Foods that are not listed in the nutritional guide are not allowed to be consumed. Some examples of such foods are given below:

1. Any canned product, be it fruits or vegetables, listed in the nutritional guide
2. Seedless fruits like grapes
3. Eggs
4. Any type of dairy product
5. Fish
6. Any type of poultry
7. Red meat
8. Soy products
9. Processed foods
10. Restaurant foods and delivered foods
11. Hybrid and fortified foods
12. Wheat
13. White sugar
14. Alcohol
15. Yeast and its products
16. Baking powder

Some other foods and ingredients have been cut off. You only need to follow the nutritional guide to know what you have to eat.

A 7-Day Alkaline Meal Plan

Among the diverse body parts, the liver is among one of the significant organs, for it has considerable capacity in body detoxification. Through this body detoxification, synthetics and other outside substances like poisons and even defecation, pee, and sweat are expelled from the body. These substances originate from the unsafe nourishments that we eat like handled and non-regular rich nourishments, liquor drinks that we devour, cigarettes that we smoke, and even drugs that we expend for anti-infection treatment and hormone elective drugs. These substances are the ones that our bodies attempt to take out every day.

When there are many harming materials inside the body, the liver needs to keep keeping up until its ability runs out. When this is dismissed, vast amounts of poisons can be gathered in the body and will cause many body issues and diseases. To anticipate this and keep up excellent health, we should experience a detoxification diet and take significant consideration of our liver.

A liver detoxification plan can be completed either on a three-day, seven-day, or twenty-one-day program. This depends on a firm focus on a diet with unprocessed and natural foods grown from the ground, entire grains, and water cure with enough measure of water or liquid other option. Nourishments that are wealthy in fat or sugar, caffeine, liquor drinks, unnatural and human-made nourishment, drugs, and low-quality nourishments would all be able to must be put to a stop, at any rate, seven days before the diet plan.

One to Three Days. This is the period to start your fluid diet plan where you need to drink around ten to twelve glasses of water ordinarily alongside frequently crushed lime juice. Even though it can indeed be challenging to execute this diet because of the weariness and slightness, light exercise can be included as a request to affix the method of flushing the poisons out of the body. Additionally, you should shun taking in any sort of milk or dairy item.

Four to Six Days. Fresh organic products, vegetables, and entire grains can be expended like celery, apples, carrots, oranges, which would all be able to be blended into one juice. The juice can incorporate your selection of leafy foods. Even though healthy nourishments are devoured, there are as yet liquid choices, for example, natural teas for around a few cups every day. Concerning suppers, they can incorporate cut and bubbled vegetables like celery, carrots, broccoli, and spinach. Besides, you can likewise utilize soups that can be taken in at regular intervals.

Seven Days. Along with the leafy foods, the liquids are expended together. They would all be able to be arranged by having them crude or steamed. Additionally, you can consume rosemary tea and dandelion options, which can be useful for this period.

You can generally change the sorts of foods grown from the ground that you will use as long as you oblige the strategy. When the seventh day is a doe, you can participate in the typical diet; finally, however, there is still a restriction on liquor consumption for around one entire week after the detoxification diet. You have to end the food once you feel torment, disorder, and squeamishness. Most likely, this detoxification diet can have an enormous impact on the advancement and support of a healthy lifestyle.

Instructions to Detox Your Body With Alternative Therapies

Conventional Chinese Medicine (TCM) is a fantastic asset when figuring out how to detox your body, and is mainly prescribed for treating stomach related issue, for example, bad-tempered inside syndrome; ceaseless skin conditions like dermatitis; weariness and despair; hormonal awkward nature, for example, PMS; endometriosis and poor sperm tally, and barrenness (both male and female). It can create results with interminable conditions that Western methods neglect to help. At the point when joined with a detox diet, it can make perceptible upgrades to a people's health and prosperity.

Self-finding and treatment of ailments are not suggested; however, at some TCM focuses, you can portray your side effects to the specialist behind the counter and get a suitable cure on the spot. TCM can be useful for treating individuals experiencing withdrawal from drug and liquor addictions. Liquor makes liver and nerve bladder uneven characters, which realizes a mix of unnecessary moistness and warmth.

Numerous drugs are prepared through the liver, making it warmed and blocked, so the liver's blood gets frail and insufficient. TCM equations center on clearing and supporting the liver and nerve bladder, while simultaneously treating the heart, to help quiet the brain and sensory system. Consolidating TCM with figuring out how to detox your body yourself is probably the best thing you can accomplish for your health.

Chapter 3: Soups

1. Creamy Avocado-Broccoli Soup

Preparation Time: 10 minutes
Cooking Time: 15 minutes
Servings: 1-2
Ingredients:

- 2-3 flowers broccoli
- 1 small avocado
- 1 yellow onion
- 1 green or red pepper
- 1 celery stalk
- 2 cups of vegetable broth (yeast-free)
- Celtic sea salt to taste

Directions:
Warm vegetable stock (don't bubble). Include hacked onion and broccoli, and warm for a few minutes. At that point, put the avocado, pepper, and celery in the blender and blend until the soup is smooth (include some more water whenever wanted). Season and serve warm. Delicious!!
Nutrition:

- Calories: 60g
- Carbohydrates: 11g
- Fat: 2 g
- Protein: 2g

2. Fresh Garden Vegetable Soup

Preparation Time: 7 minutes
Cooking Time: 20 minutes
Servings: 1-2
Ingredients:

- 2 huge carrots
- 1 little zucchini
- 1 celery stem
- 1 cup of broccoli
- 3 stalks of asparagus
- 1 yellow onion
- 1 quart of (antacid) water
- 4-5 tsps. of sans yeast vegetable stock
- 1 tsp. new basil
- 2 tsps. Ocean salt to taste

Directions:

1. Put water in a pot, include the vegetable stock just as the onion and boil it.
2. In the meantime, cleave the zucchini, the broccoli, and the asparagus, and shred the carrots and the celery stem in a food processor.
3. When the water is bubbling, it would be ideal if you turn off the oven as we would prefer not to heat up the vegetables. Simply put them all in the high temp water and hold up until the vegetables arrive at wanted delicacy.
4. Permit to cool somewhat, at that point put all fixings into a blender and blend until you get a thick, smooth consistency.

Nutrition:

- Calories: 43
- Carbohydrates: 7g
- Fat: 1 g

3. Rawsome Gazpacho Soup

Preparation Time: 7 minutes
Cooking Time: 3 hours
Servings: 3-4
Ingredients:

- 500g tomatoes
- 1 small cucumber
- 1 red pepper
- 1 onion
- 2 cloves of garlic
- 1 small chili

- 1 quart of water (preferably alkaline water)
- 4 tbsp. cold-pressed olive oil
- Juice of one fresh lemon
- 1 dash of cayenne pepper
- Sea salt to taste

Directions:

1. Remove the skin of the cucumber and cut all vegetables in large pieces.
2. Put all ingredients except the olive oil in a blender and mix until smooth.
3. Add the olive oil and mix again until oil is emulsified.
4. Put the soup in the fridge and chill for at least 2 hours (soup should be served ice cold).
5. Add some salt and pepper to taste, mix, place the soup in bowls, garnish with chopped scallions, cucumbers, tomatoes, and peppers and enjoy!

Nutrition:

- Calories: 39
- Carbohydrates: 8g
- Fat: 0.5 g
- Protein: 0.2g

4. Alkaline Carrot Soup with Fresh Mushrooms

Preparation Time: 10 minutes
Cooking Time: 20 minutes
Servings: 1-2
Ingredients:

- 4 mid-sized carrots
- 4 mid-sized potatoes
- 10 enormous new mushrooms (champignons or chanterelles)
- 1/2 white onion
- 2 tbsp. olive oil (cold squeezed, additional virgin)
- 3 cups vegetable stock
- 2 tbsp. parsley, new and cleaved
- Salt and new white pepper

Directions:

1. Wash and strip carrots and potatoes and dice them.
2. Warm up vegetable stock in a pot on medium heat. Cook carrots and potatoes for around 15 minutes. Meanwhile finely shape onion and braise them in a container with olive oil for around 3 minutes.
3. Wash mushrooms, slice them to wanted size, and add to the container, cooking for an additional of approximately 5 minutes, blending at times. Blend carrots, vegetable stock and potatoes, and put the substance of the skillet into the pot.
4. When nearly done, season with parsley, salt, and pepper and serve hot. Appreciate this alkalizing soup!

Nutrition:

- Calories: 75
- Carbohydrates: 13g
- Fat: 1.8g
- Protein: 1 g

5. Swiss Cauliflower-Soup

Preparation Time: 10 minutes
Cooking Time: 15 minutes
Servings: 3-4
Ingredients:

- 2 cups cauliflower pieces
- 1 cup potatoes, cubed
- 2 cups vegetable stock (without yeast)
- 2 tbsp. new chives
- 1 tbsp. pumpkin seeds
- 1 touch of nutmeg and cayenne pepper

Directions:

1. Cook cauliflower and potato in vegetable stock until delicate and blend it.
2. Season the soup with nutmeg and cayenne, and possibly somewhat salt and pepper.
3. Optionally, include some creamy vegan cheese and mix a couple of moments until the soup is smooth and prepared to serve. Enhance it with pumpkin seeds.

Nutrition:

- Calories: 65
- Carbohydrates: 13g
- Fat: 2g
- Protein: 1g

6. Chilled Parsley-Gazpacho with Lime & Cucumber

Preparation Time: 10 minutes
Cooking Time: 2 hours
Servings: 1
Ingredients:

- 4-5 middle-sized tomatoes
- 2 tbsp. olive oil, extra virgin, and cold-pressed
- 2 large cups fresh parsley
- 2 ripe avocados
- 2 cloves garlic, diced
- 2 limes, juiced
- 4 cups vegetable broth
- 1 middle-sized cucumber
- 2 small red onions, diced
- 1 tsp. dried oregano
- 1½ tsp. paprika powder
- ½ tsp. cayenne pepper
- Sea salt and freshly ground pepper to taste

Directions:

1. In a pan, heat up olive oil and sauté onions and garlic until translucent. Set aside to cool down.
2. Use a large blender and blend parsley, avocado, tomatoes, cucumber, vegetable broth, lime juice, and onion-garlic mix until smooth. Add some water if desired, and season with cayenne pepper, paprika powder, oregano, salt, and pepper. Blend again and put in the fridge for at least 1, 5 hours.
   Tip: Add chives or dill to the gazpacho. Enjoy this great alkaline (cold) soup!

Nutrition:

- Calories: 48
- Carbohydrates: 12 g
- Fat: 0.8g

7. Chilled Avocado Tomato Soup

Preparation Time: 7 minutes
Cooking Time: 20 minutes
Servings: 1-2
Ingredients:

- 2 small avocados
- 2 large tomatoes
- 1 stalk of celery
- 1 small onion
- 1 clove of garlic
- Juice of 1 fresh lemon
- 1 cup of water (best: alkaline water)
- A handful of fresh lavage
- Parsley and sea salt to taste

Directions:

1. Scoop the avocados and cut all veggies in little pieces.
2. Spot all fixings in a blender and blend until smooth.
3. Serve chilled and appreciate this nutritious and sound soluble soup

formula!

Nutrition:

- Calories: 68
- Carbohydrates: 15g
- Fat: 2g
- Protein: .8g

8. Pumpkin and White Bean Soup with Sage

Preparation Time: 10 minutes
Cooking Time: 40 minutes
Servings: 3-4
Ingredients:

- 1 ½ pound pumpkin
- ½ pound yams
- ½ pound white beans
- 1 onion
- 2 cloves of garlic
- 1 tbsp. of cold squeezed additional virgin olive oil
- 1 tbsp. of spices (your top picks)
- 1 tbsp. of sage
- 1 ½ quart water (best: antacid water)
- A spot of ocean salt and pepper

Directions:

1. Cut the pumpkin and potatoes in shapes, cut the onion and cut the garlic, the spices, and the sage in fine pieces.
2. Sauté the onion and also the garlic in olive oil for around two or three minutes.
3. Include the potatoes, pumpkin, spices, and sage and fry for an additional 5 minutes.
4. At that point include the water and cook for around 30 minutes (spread the pot with a top) until vegetables are delicate.
5. At long last include the beans and some salt and pepper. Cook for an additional 5 minutes and serve right away. Prepared!! Appreciate this antacid soup. Alkalizing tasty!

Nutrition:

- Calories: 78
- Carbohydrates: 12g

9. Alkaline Carrot Soup With Millet

Preparation Time: 7 minutes
Cooking Time: 40 minutes
Servings: 3-4
Ingredients:

- 2 cups cauliflower pieces
- 1 cup potatoes, cubed
- 2 cups vegetable stock (without yeast)
- Vegan cheese
- 2 tbsp. new chives
- 1 tbsp. pumpkin seeds
- 1 touch of nutmeg and cayenne pepper

Directions:

1. Cook cauliflower and potato in vegetable stock until delicate and blend it.
2. Season the soup with nutmeg and cayenne, and possibly somewhat salt and pepper.
3. Include the vegan cheese and chives and mix a couple of moments until the soup is smooth and prepared to serve. It can be enhanced with pumpkin seeds.

Nutrition:

- Calories: 65
- Carbohydrates: 15g
- Fat: 1g
- Protein: 2g

10. Alkaline Pumpkin Tomato Soup

Preparation Time: 15 minutes
Cooking Time: 30 minutes
Servings: 3-4
Ingredients:

- 1 quart of water (if accessible: soluble water)
- 400g new tomatoes, stripped and diced
- 1 medium-sized sweet pumpkin
- 5 yellow onions
- 1 tbsp. cold squeezed additional virgin olive oil
- 2 tsp. ocean salt or natural salt
- Touch of cayenne pepper
- Your preferred spices (discretionary)
- Bunch of new parsley

Directions:

1. Cut onions in little pieces and sauté with some oil in a significant pot.
2. Cut the pumpkin down the middle, at that point remove the stem and scoop out the seeds.
3. At long last scoop out the fragile living creature and put it in the pot.
4. Include likewise the tomatoes and the water and cook for around 20 minutes.
5. At that point empty the soup into a food processor and blend well for a couple of moments. Sprinkle with salt pepper and other spices.
6. Fill bowls and trimming with new parsley. Make the most of your alkalizing soup!

Nutrition:

- Calories: 78
- Carbohydrates: 20
- Fat: 0.5g
- Protein: 1.5g

11. Alkaline Pumpkin Coconut Soup

Preparation Time: 10 minutes
Cooking Time: 15 minutes
Servings: 3-4
Ingredients:

- 2lb pumpkin
- 6 cups of water (best: soluble water delivered with a water ionizer)
- 1 cup low-fat coconut milk
- 5 ounces of potatoes
- 2 major onions
- 3 ounces leek
- 1 bunch of new parsley
- 1 touch of nutmeg
- 1 touch of cayenne pepper
- 1 tsp. ocean salt or natural salt
- 4 tbsp. cold squeezed additional virgin olive oil

Directions:

1. As a matter of first significance: cut the onions, the pumpkin, and the potatoes just as the hole into little pieces.
2. At that point, heat the olive oil in a significant pot and sauté the onions for a couple of moments.
3. At that point, include the water and heat up the pumpkin, potatoes, and the leek until delicate.
4. Include coconut milk.
5. Presently utilize a hand blender and puree for around 1 moment. The soup should turn out to be extremely velvety.
6. Season with salt, pepper, and nutmeg. Lastly, include the parsley and appreciate this alkalizing pumpkin soup hot or cold!

Nutrition:

- Calories: 88
- Carbohydrates: 23g
- Fat: 2.5 g
- Protein: 1.8g

12.Cold Cauliflower-Coconut Soup

Preparation Time: 7 minutes
Cooking Time: 20 minutes
Servings: 3-4
Ingredients:

- 1 pound (450g) new cauliflower
- 1 ¼ cup (300ml) unsweetened coconut milk
- 1 cup of water (best: antacid water)
- 2 tbsp. new lime juice
- 1/3 cup cold squeezed additional virgin olive oil
- 1 cup new coriander leaves, slashed
- Spot of salt and cayenne pepper
- 1 bunch of unsweetened coconut chips

Directions:

1. Steam cauliflower for around 10 minutes.
2. At that point, set up the cauliflower with coconut milk and water in a food processor and get it started until extremely smooth.
3. Include new lime squeeze, salt and pepper, a large portion of the cleaved coriander, and the oil and blend for an additional couple of moments.
4. Pour in soup bowls and embellishment with coriander and coconut chips. Appreciate!

Nutrition:

- Calories: 65
- Carbohydrates: 11g
- Fat: 0.3g
- Protein: 1.5g

13. Raw Avocado-Broccoli Soup With Cashew Nuts

Preparation Time: 10 minutes
Cooking Time: 30 minutes
Servings: 1-2
Ingredients:

- ½ cup of water (if available: alkaline water)
- ½ avocado
- 1 cup chopped broccoli
- ½ cup cashew nuts
- ½ cup alfalfa sprouts
- 1 clove of garlic
- 1 tbsp. cold-pressed extra virgin olive oil
- 1 pinch of sea salt and pepper
- Some parsley to garnish

Directions:

1. Put the cashew nuts in a blender or food processor, include some water and puree for a couple of moments.
2. Include the various fixings (except for the avocado) individually and puree each an ideal opportunity for a couple of moments.
3. Dispense the soup in a container and warm it up to the normal room temperature. Enhance with salt and pepper. In the interim dice the avocado and slash the parsley.
4. Dispense the soup in a container or plate; include the avocado dices and embellishment with parsley.
5. That's it! Enjoy this excellent healthy soup!

Nutrition:

- Calories: 48
- Carbohydrates: 18g
- Fat: 3g
- Protein: 1.4g

14.Lemon-Tarragon Soup

Preparation Time: 10 minutes
Cooking Time: 10 minutes
Servings: 1-2

Cashews and coconut milk replace heavy cream in this healthy version of the lemon-tarragon soup, balanced by tart freshly squeezed lemon juice and fragrant tarragon. It's a light, airy soup that you won't want to miss.

Ingredients:

- 1 tablespoon avocado oil
- ½ cup diced onion
- 3 garlic cloves, crushed
- ¼ plus ⅛ teaspoon sea salt
- ¼ plus ⅛ teaspoon freshly ground black pepper
- 1 (13.5-ounce) can full-fat coconut milk
- 1 tablespoon freshly squeezed lemon juice
- ½ cup raw cashews
- 1 celery stalk
- 2 tablespoons chopped fresh tarragon

Directions:

1. In a medium skillet over medium-high warmth, heat the avocado oil. Add the onion, garlic, salt, and pepper, and sauté for 3 to 5 minutes or until the onion is soft.
2. In a high-speed blender, blend the coconut milk, lemon juice, cashews, celery, and tarragon with the onion mixture until smooth. Adjust seasonings, if necessary.
3. Fill 1 huge or 2 little dishes and enjoy immediately, or transfer to a medium saucepan and warm on low heat for 3 to 5 minutes before serving.

Nutrition:

- Calories: 60
- Carbohydrates: 13 g
- Protein: 0.8 g

15.Chilled Cucumber and Lime Soup

Preparation Time: 5 minutes
Cooking Time: 20 minutes
Servings: 1-2

Chilled soups are perfect for the hot summer months, and this easy soup is made with garden fresh vegetables with no cooking involved. Simply prepare the veggies, add them to a blender, and lunch is served!

Ingredients:

- 1 cucumber, peeled
- ½ zucchini, peeled
- 1 tablespoon freshly squeezed lime juice
- 1 tablespoon fresh cilantro leaves
- 1 garlic clove, crushed
- ¼ teaspoon of sea salt

Directions:

1. In a blender, blend the cucumber, zucchini, lime juice, cilantro, garlic, and salt until well combined. Add more salt, if necessary.
2. Fill 1 huge or 2 little dishes and enjoy immediately, or refrigerate for 15 to 20 minutes to chill before serving.

Nutrition:

- Calories: 48
- Carbohydrates: 8 g
- Fat: 1g
- Protein: .5g

16.Coconut, Cilantro, and Jalapeño Soup

Preparation Time: 5 minutes
Cooking Time: 5 minutes
Servings: 1-2

This soup is a nutrient dream. Cilantro is a natural anti-inflammatory and is also excellent for detoxification. And one single jalapeño has an entire day's worth of vitamin C!

Ingredients:

- 2 tablespoons avocado oil
- ½ cup diced onions
- 3 garlic cloves, crushed
- ¼ teaspoon of sea salt
- 1 (13.5-ounce) can full-fat coconut milk
- 1 tablespoon freshly squeezed lime juice
- ½ to 1 jalapeño
- 2 tablespoons fresh cilantro leaves

Directions:

1. In a medium skillet over medium-high warmth, heat the avocado oil. Include the garlic, onion salt, and pepper, and sauté for 3 to 5 minutes, or until the onions are soft.
2. In a blender, blend the coconut milk, lime juice, jalapeño, and cilantro with the onion mixture until creamy.
3. Fill 1 huge or 2 little dishes and enjoy it.

Nutrition:

- Calories: 75
- Carbohydrates: 13 g
- Fat: 2 g
- Protein: 4 g

17. Spicy Watermelon Gazpacho

Preparation Time: 5 minutes
Cooking Time: 5 minutes
Servings: 1-2

At first taste, this soup may have you wondering if you're lunching on a hot and spicy salsa. It has the heat and seasonings of a traditional tomato-based salsa, but it also has a faint sweetness from the cool watermelon. The soup is really hot with a whole jalapeño, so if you don't like food too hot, just use half a jalapeño.

Ingredients:

- 2 cups cubed watermelon
- ¼ cup diced onion
- ¼ cup packed cilantro leaves
- ½ to 1 jalapeño
- 2 tablespoons freshly squeezed lime juice

Directions:

1. In a blender or food processor, pulse to combine the watermelon, onion, cilantro, jalapeño, and lime juice only long enough to break down the ingredients, leaving them very finely diced and taking care to not over process.
2. Pour into 1 large or 2 small bowls and enjoy.

Nutrition:

- Calories: 35
- Carbohydrates: 12
- Fat: .4 g

18. Roasted Carrot and Leek Soup

Preparation Time: 4 minutes
Cooking Time: 30 minutes
Servings: 3-4

The carrot, a root vegetable, is an excellent source of antioxidants (1 cup has 113 percent of your daily value of vitamin A), and fibre (1 cup has 14 percent of your daily value). This bright and colourful soup freezes well to enjoy later when you're short on time.

Ingredients:

- 6 carrots
- 1 cup chopped onion
- 1 fennel bulb, cubed

- 2 garlic cloves, crushed
- 2 tablespoons avocado oil
- 1 teaspoon of sea salt
- 1 teaspoon freshly ground black pepper
- 2 cups almond milk, plus more if desired

Directions:

1. Preheat the oven to 400°F. Line a baking sheet with parchment paper.
2. Cut the carrots into thirds, and then cut each third in half. Transfer to a medium bowl.
3. Add the onion, fennel, garlic, and avocado oil, and toss to coat. Season with the salt and pepper, and toss again.
4. Transfer the vegetables to the prepared baking sheet, and roast for 30 minutes.
5. Remove from the oven and allow the vegetables to cool.
6. In a high-speed blender, blend the almond milk and roasted vegetables until creamy and smooth. Adjust the seasonings, if necessary, and add additional milk if you prefer a thinner consistency.
7. Pour into 2 large or 4 small bowls and enjoy.

Nutrition:

- Calories: 55
- Carbohydrates: 12g
- Fat: 1.5 g
- Protein: 1.8 g

19.Creamy Lentil and Potato Stew

Preparation Time: 10 minutes
Cooking Time: 30 minutes
Servings: 4

This is a hearty stew that is sure to be a favourite. It's a one-pot meal that is the perfect comfort food. With fresh vegetables and herbs along with protein-rich lentils, it's both healthy and filling. Any lentil variety would work, even a mixed, sprouted lentil blend. Another bonus of this recipe: It's freezer-friendly.

Ingredients:

- 2 tablespoons avocado oil
- ½ cup diced onion
- 2 garlic cloves, crushed
- 1 to 1½ teaspoons of sea salt
- 1 teaspoon freshly ground black pepper
- 1 cup dry lentils
- 2 carrots, sliced
- 1 cup peeled and cubed potato
- 1 celery stalk, diced
- 2 fresh oregano sprigs, chopped
- 2 fresh tarragon sprigs, chopped
- 5 cups vegetable broth, divided
- 1 (13.5-ounce) can full-fat coconut milk

Directions:

1. In a great soup pot over average-high hotness, heat the avocado oil. Include the garlic, onion, salt, and pepper, and sauté for 3 to 5 minutes, or until the onion is soft.
2. Add the lentils, carrots, potato, celery, oregano, tarragon, and 2½ cups of vegetable broth, and stir.
3. Get to a boil, decrease the heat to medium-low, and cook, stirring frequently and adding additional vegetable broth a half cup at a time to make sure there is enough liquid for the lentils and potatoes to cook, for 20 to 25 minutes, or until the potatoes and lentils are soft.
4. Take away from the heat, and stir in

the coconut milk. Pour into 4 soup bowls and enjoy.

Nutrition:

- Calories: 85
- Carbohydrates: 20g
- Fat: 3g
- Protein: 3g

20. Roasted Garlic and Cauliflower Soup

Preparation Time: 10 minutes
Cooking Time: 35 minutes
Servings: 1-2

Roasted garlic is always a treat, and paired with cauliflower in this wonderful soup, what you get is a deeply satisfying soup with savoury, rustic flavors. Blended, the result is a smooth, thick, and creamy soup, but if you prefer a thinner consistency, just add a little more vegetable broth to thin it out. Cauliflower is anti-inflammatory, high in antioxidants, and a good source of vitamin C (1 cup has 86 percent of your daily value).

Ingredients:

- 4 cups bite-size cauliflower florets
- 5 garlic cloves
- 1½ tablespoons avocado oil
- ¾ teaspoon of sea salt
- ½ teaspoon freshly ground black pepper
- 1 cup almond milk
- 1 cup vegetable broth, plus more if desired

Directions:

1. Preheat the oven to 450°F. Line a baking sheet with parchment paper.
2. In a medium bowl, toss the cauliflower and garlic with the avocado oil to coat. Season with the salt and pepper, and toss again.
3. Transfer to the prepared baking sheet and roast for 30 minutes. Cool before adding to the blender.
4. In a high-speed blender, blend the cooled vegetables, almond milk, and vegetable broth until creamy and smooth. Adjust the salt and pepper, if necessary, and add additional vegetable broth if you prefer a thinner consistency.
5. Transfer to a medium saucepan, and lightly warm on medium-low heat for 3 to 5 minutes.
6. Ladle into 1 large or 2 small bowls and enjoy.

Nutrition:

- Calories: 48
- Carbohydrates: 11g
- Protein: 1.5g

21. Beefless "Beef" Stew

Preparation Time: 10 minutes
Cooking Time: 0 minutes
Servings: 4

The potatoes, carrots, aromatics, and herbs in this soup meld so well together, you'll forget there's typically beef in this stew. Hearty and flavourful, this one-pot comfort food is perfect for a fall or winter dinner.

Ingredients:

- 1 tablespoon avocado oil
- 1 cup onion, diced
- 2 garlic cloves, crushed
- 1 teaspoon of sea salt
- 1 teaspoon freshly ground black pepper
- 3 cups vegetable broth, plus more if desired
- 2 cups water, plus more if desired
- 3 cups sliced carrot
- 1 large potato, cubed
- 2 celery stalks, diced

- 1 teaspoon dried oregano
- 1 dried bay leaf

Directions:

1. In a medium soup pot over medium heat, heat the avocado oil. Include the onion, garlic, salt, and pepper, and sauté for 2 to 3 minutes, or until the onion is soft.
2. Add the vegetable broth, water, carrot, potato, celery, oregano, and bay leaf, and stir. Get to a boil, decrease the heat to medium-low, and cook for 30 to 45 minutes, or until the potatoes and carrots are soft.
3. Adjust the seasonings, if necessary, and add additional water or vegetable broth, if a soupier consistency is preferred, in half-cup increments.
4. Ladle into 4 soup bowls and enjoy.

Nutrition:

- Calories: 59
- Carbohydrates: 12g

22. Creamy Mushroom Soup

Preparation Time: 5 minutes
Cooking Time: 20 minutes
Servings: 4

This savoury, earthy soup is a must-try if you love mushrooms. Shiitake and baby Portobello (cremini) mushrooms are used here, but you can substitute them with your favourite mushroom varieties. Full-fat coconut milk gives it that close-your-eyes-and-savor-it creaminess that pushes the soup into the comfort food realm—perfect for those cold evenings when you need a warm soup to heat up your insides.

Ingredients:

- 1 tablespoon avocado oil
- 1 cup sliced shiitake mushrooms
- 1 cup sliced cremini mushrooms
- 1 cup diced onion
- 1 garlic clove, crushed
- 3/4 teaspoon of sea salt
- 1/2 teaspoon freshly ground black pepper
- 1 cup vegetable broth
- 1 (13.5-ounce) can full-fat coconut milk
- 1/2 teaspoon dried thyme
- 1 tablespoon coconut aminos

Directions:

1. In a great soup pot over average-high hotness, heat the avocado oil. Add the mushrooms, onion, garlic, salt, and pepper, and sauté for 2 to 3 minutes, or until the onion is soft.
2. Add the vegetable broth, coconut milk, thyme, and coconut aminos. Reduce the heat to medium-low, and simmer for about 15 minutes, stirring occasionally.
3. Adjust seasonings, if necessary, ladle into 2 large or 4 small bowls, and enjoy.

Nutrition:

- Calories: 65
- Carbohydrates: 12g
- Fat: 2g
- Protein: 2g

23. Chilled Berry and Mint Soup

Preparation Time: 5 minutes
Cooking Time: 20 minutes
Servings: 1-2

There's no better way to cool down when it's hot outside than with this chilled, sweet mixed berry soup. It's light and showcases summer's berry bounty: raspberries, blackberries, and blueberries. The fresh mint brightens the soup and keeps the sweetness in check. This soup isn't just for lunch or dinner—you can try it as a quick breakfast, too! If you like a thinner consistency for this, just add a little extra water.

Ingredients:

FOR THE SWEETENER

- ¼ cup unrefined whole cane sugar, such as Sucanat
- ¼ cup water, plus more if desired

FOR THE SOUP

- 1 cup of mixed berries (raspberries, blackberries, blueberries)
- ½ cup of water
- 1 teaspoon freshly squeezed lemon juice
- 8 fresh mint leaves

Directions:

To prepare the sweetener

1. In a small saucepan over medium-low, heat the sugar and water, stirring continuously for 1 to 2 minutes, until the sugar is dissolved. Cool.

To prepare the soup

1. In a blender, blend the cooled sugar water with the berries, water, lemon juice, and mint leaves until well combined.
2. Transfer the mixture to the refrigerator and allow chilling completely, about 20 minutes.
3. Ladle into 1 large or 2 small bowls and enjoy.

Nutrition:

- Calories: 89
- Carbohydrates: 12g
- Fat: 6g
- Protein: 2.2 g

24. White Bean Soup

Preparation Time: 10 minutes
Cooking Time: 40 minutes
Servings: 6

Ingredients:

- 2 cups white beans, rinsed
- ¼ tsp. cayenne pepper
- 1 tsp. dried oregano
- ½ tsp. fresh rosemary, chopped
- 3 cups filtered alkaline water
- 3 cups unsweetened almond milk
- 3 garlic cloves, minced
- 2 celery stalks, diced
- 1 onion, chopped
- 1 tbsp. olive oil
- ½ tsp. sea salt

Directions:

1. Add oil into the instant pot and set the pot on sauté mode.
2. Add carrots, celery, and onion in oil and sauté until softened, about 5 minutes.
3. Add garlic and sauté for a minute.
4. Add beans, seasonings, water, and almond milk and stir to combine.
5. Cover pot with lid and cook on high pressure for 35 minutes.
6. When finished, release pressure naturally, then open the lid.
7. Stir well and serve.

Nutrition:

- Calories 276
- Fat 4.8 g
- Carbohydrates 44.2 g
- Sugar 2.3 g
- Protein 16.6 g
- Cholesterol 0 mg

25. Kale Cauliflower Soup

Preparation Time: 10 minutes
Cooking Time: 25 minutes
Servings: 4

Ingredients:

- 2 cups baby kale

- ½ cup unsweetened coconut milk
- 4 cups of water
- 1 large cauliflower head, chopped
- 3 garlic cloves, peeled
- 2 carrots, peeled and chopped
- 2 onion, chopped
- 3 tbsp. olive oil
- Pepper
- Salt

Directions:

1. Add oil into the instant pot and set the pot on sauté mode.
2. Add carrot, garlic, and onion to the pot and sauté for 5-7 minutes.
3. Add water and cauliflower and stir well.
4. Cover pot with lid and cook on high pressure for 20 minutes.
5. When finished, release pressure using the quick release, then open the lid.
6. Add kale and coconut milk and stir well.
7. Blend the soup utilizing a submersion blender until smooth.
8. Season with pepper and salt.

Nutrition:

- Calories 261
- Fat 18.1 g
- Carbohydrates 23.9 g
- Sugar 9.9 g
- Protein 6.6 g
- Cholesterol 0 mg

26. Healthy Broccoli Asparagus Soup

Preparation Time: 10 minutes
Cooking Time: 20 minutes
Servings: 6
Ingredients:

- 2 cups broccoli florets, chopped
- 15 asparagus spears, ends trimmed and chopped
- 1 tsp. dried oregano
- 1 tbsp. fresh thyme leaves
- ½ cup unsweetened almond milk
- 3 ½ cups filtered alkaline water
- 2 cups cauliflower florets, chopped
- 2 tsp. garlic, chopped
- 1 cup onion, chopped
- 2 tbsp. olive oil
- Pepper
- Salt

Directions:

1. Add oil in the instant pot and set the pot on sauté mode.
2. Add onion to the olive oil and sauté until onion is softened.
3. Add garlic and sauté for 30 seconds.
4. Add all vegetables and water and stir well.
5. Cover pot with lid and cook on manual mode for 3 minutes.
6. When finished, release pressure naturally, then open the lid.
7. Blend the soup utilizing a submersion blender until smooth.
8. Stir in almond milk, herbs, pepper, and salt.
9. Serve and enjoy.

Nutrition:

- Calories 85
- Fat 5.2 g
- Carbohydrates 8.8 g
- Sugar 3.3 g
- Protein 3.3 g
- Cholesterol 0 mg

27. Creamy Asparagus Soup

Preparation Time: 10 minutes
Cooking Time: 30 minutes
Servings: 6
Ingredients:

- 2 lbs. fresh asparagus cut off woody stems
- ¼ tsp. lime zest
- 2 tbsp. lime juice
- 14 oz. coconut milk
- 1 tsp. dried thyme
- ½ tsp. oregano
- ½ tsp. sage
- 1 ½ cups filtered alkaline water
- 1 cauliflower head, cut into florets
- 1 tbsp. garlic, minced
- 1 leek, sliced
- 3 tbsp. coconut oil
- Pinch of Himalayan salt

Directions:

1. Preheat the oven to 400 F/ 200 C.
2. Line baking tray with parchment paper and set aside.
3. Arrange asparagus spears on a baking tray. Drizzle with 2 tablespoons of coconut oil and sprinkle with salt, thyme, oregano, and sage.
4. Bake in preheated oven for 20-25 minutes.
5. Add remaining oil in the instant pot and set the pot on sauté mode.
6. Put some garlic and leek to the pot and sauté for 2-3 minutes.
7. Add cauliflower florets and water in the pot and stir well.
8. Cover pot with a lid and select steam mode and set timer for 4 minutes.
9. When finished, release pressure using the quick release.
10. Add roasted asparagus, lime zest, lime juice, and coconut milk and stir well.
11. Blend the soup utilizing a submersion blender until smooth.
12. Serve and enjoy.

Nutrition:

- Calories 265
- Fat 22.9 g
- Carbohydrates 14.7 g
- Sugar 6.7 g
- Protein 6.1 g
- Cholesterol 0 mg

28. Quick Broccoli Soup

Preparation Time: 5 minutes
Cooking Time: 10 minutes
Servings: 6
Ingredients:

- 1 lb. broccoli, chopped
- 6 cups filtered alkaline water
- 1 onion, diced
- 2 tbsp. olive oil
- Pepper
- Salt

Directions:

1. Add oil into the instant pot and set the pot on sauté mode.
2. Add the onion in olive oil and sauté until softened.
3. Add broccoli and water and stir well.
4. Cover pot with top and cook on manual high pressure for 3 minutes.
5. When finished, release pressure using the quick release, and then open the lid.
6. Blend the soup utilizing a submersion blender until smooth.
7. Season soup with pepper and salt.
8. Serve and enjoy.

Nutrition:

- Calories 73
- Fat 4.9 g

- Carbohydrates 6.7 g
- Protein 2.3 g
- Sugar 2.1 g
- Cholesterol 0 mg

29. Green Lentil Soup

Preparation Time: 10 minutes
Cooking Time: 30 minutes
Servings: 4
Ingredients:

- 1 ½ cups green lentils, rinsed
- 4 cups baby spinach
- 4 cups filtered alkaline water
- 1 tsp. Italian seasoning
- 2 tsp. fresh thyme
- 14 oz. tomatoes, diced
- 3 garlic cloves, minced
- 2 celery stalks, chopped
- 1 carrot, chopped
- 1 onion, chopped
- Pepper
- Sea salt

Directions:

1. Add all ingredients except spinach into the direct pot and mix fine.
2. Cover pot with top and cook on manual high pressure for 18 minutes.
3. When finished, release pressure using the quick release, and then open the lid.
4. Add spinach and stir well.
5. Serve and enjoy.

Nutrition:

- Calories 306
- Fat 1.5 g
- Carbohydrates 53.7 g
- Sugar 6.4 g
- Protein 21 g
- Cholesterol 1 mg

30. Squash Soup

Preparation Time: 10 minutes
Cooking Time: 40 minutes
Servings: 4
Ingredients:

- 3 lbs. butternut squash, peeled and cubed
- 1 tbsp. curry powder
- 1/2 cup unsweetened coconut milk
- 3 cups filtered alkaline water
- 2 garlic cloves, minced
- 1 large onion, minced
- 1 tsp. olive oil

Directions:

1. Add olive oil in the instant pot and set the pot on sauté mode.
2. Add onion and cook until tender, about 8 minutes.
3. Add curry powder and garlic and sauté for a minute.
4. Add butternut squash, water, and salt and stir well.
5. Cover pot with lid and cook on soup mode for 30 minutes.
6. When finished, release pressure naturally for 10 minutes, then release using the quick release, and then open the lid.
7. Blend the soup utilizing a submersion blender until smooth.
8. Add coconut milk and stir well.
9. Serve warm and enjoy.

Nutrition:

- Calories 254
- Fat 8.9 g
- Carbohydrates 46.4 g
- Sugar 10.1 g
- Protein 4.8 g
- Cholesterol 0 mg

31.Tomato Soup

Preparation Time: 5 minutes
Cooking Time: 20 minutes
Servings: 4
Ingredients:

- 6 tomatoes, chopped
- 1 onion, diced
- 14 oz. coconut milk
- 1 tsp. turmeric
- 1 tsp. garlic, minced
- 1/4 cup cilantro, chopped
- 1/2 tsp. cayenne pepper
- 1 tsp. ginger, minced
- 1/2 tsp. sea salt

Directions:

1. Add all ingredients to the direct pot and mix fine.
2. Cover the instant pot with a lid and cook on manual high pressure for 5 minutes.
3. When finished, release pressure naturally for 10 minutes then release using the quick release.
4. Blend the soup utilizing a submersion blender until smooth.
5. Stir well and serve.

Nutrition:

- Calories 81
- Fat 3.5 g
- Carbohydrates 11.6 g
- Sugar 6.1 g
- Protein 2.5 g
- Cholesterol 0 mg

32. Basil Zucchini Soup

Preparation Time: 10 minutes
Cooking Time: 20 minutes
Servings: 4
Ingredients:

- 3 medium zucchinis, peeled and chopped
- 1/4 cup basil, chopped
- 1 large leek, chopped
- 3 cups filtered alkaline water
- 1 tbsp. lemon juice
- 3 tbsp. olive oil
- 2 tsp. sea salt

Directions:

1. Add 2 tbsp. oil into the pot and set the pot on sauté mode.
2. Add zucchini and sauté for 5 minutes.
3. Add basil and leeks and sauté for 2-3 minutes.
4. Add lemon juice, water, and salt. Stir well.
5. Cover pot with lid and cook on high pressure for 8 minutes.
6. When finished, release pressure naturally, then open the lid.
7. Blend the soup utilizing a submersion blender until smooth.
8. Top with remaining olive oil and serve.

Nutrition:

- Calories 157
- Fat 11.9 g
- Carbohydrates 8.9 g
- Protein 5.8 g
- Sugar 4 g
- Cholesterol 0 mg

33. Summer Vegetable Soup

Preparation Time: 5 minutes
Cooking Time: 20 minutes
Servings: 10
Ingredients:

- 1/2 cup basil, chopped
- 2 bell peppers, seeded and sliced
- 1/ cup green beans, trimmed and cut into pieces
- 8 cups filtered alkaline water

- 1 medium summer squash, sliced
- 1 medium zucchini, sliced
- 2 large tomatoes, sliced
- 1 small eggplant, sliced
- 6 garlic cloves, smashed
- 1 medium onion, diced
- Pepper
- Salt

Directions:

1. Combine all elements into the direct pot and mix fine.
2. Cover pot with lid and cook on soup mode for 10 minutes.
3. Release pressure using the quick release, then open the lid.
4. Blend the soup utilizing a submersion blender until smooth.
5. Serve and enjoy.

Nutrition:

- Calories 84
- Fat 1.6 g
- Carbohydrates 12.8 g
- Protein 6.1 g
- Sugar 6.1 g
- Cholesterol 0 mg

34. Spicy Carrot Soup

Preparation Time: 10 minutes
Cooking Time: 20 minutes
Servings: 6
Ingredients:

- 8 large carrots, peeled and chopped
- 1 1/2 cups filtered alkaline water
- 14 oz. coconut milk
- 3 garlic cloves, peeled
- 1 tbsp. red curry paste
- 1/4 cup olive oil
- 1 onion, chopped
- Salt

Directions:

1. Combine all elements into the direct pot and mix fine.
2. Cover the pot with a lid, select the manual, and set the timer for 15 minutes.
3. Release pressure naturally, then open the lid.
4. Blend the soup utilizing a submersion blender until smooth.
5. Serve and enjoy.

Nutrition:

- Calories 267
- Fat 22 g
- Carbohydrates 13 g
- Protein 4 g
- Sugar 5 g
- Cholesterol 20 mg

35. Zucchini Soup

Preparation Time: 10 minutes
Cooking Time: 30 minutes
Servings: 10
Ingredients:

- 10 cups zucchini, chopped
- 32 oz. filtered alkaline water
- 13.5 oz. coconut milk
- 1 tbsp. Thai curry paste

Directions:

1. Combine all elements into the direct pot and mix fine.
2. Cover pot with lid and cook on manual high pressure for 10 minutes.
3. Release pressure using the quick release, then open the lid.
4. Use a blender to blend the soup until smooth.
5. Serve and enjoy.

Nutrition:

- Calories 122
- Fat 9.8 g

- Carbohydrates 6.6 g
- Protein 4.1 g
- Sugar 3.6 g
- Cholesterol 0 mg

36. Dill Celery Soup

Preparation Time: 10 minutes
Cooking Time: 30 minutes
Servings: 4
Ingredients:

- 6 cups celery stalk, chopped
- 2 cups filtered alkaline water
- 1 medium onion, chopped
- 1/2 tsp. dill
- 1 cup of coconut milk
- 1/4 tsp. sea salt

Directions:

1. Combine all elements into the direct pot and mix fine.
2. Cover pot with a lid and select soup mode; it takes 30 minutes.
3. Release pressure using the quick release, then open the lid carefully.
4. Blend the soup utilizing a submersion blender until smooth.
5. Stir well and serve.

Nutrition:

- Calories 193
- Fat 15.3 g
- Carbohydrates 10.9 g
- Protein 5.2 g
- Sugar 5.6 g
- Cholesterol 0 mg

Chapter 4: Salads

37. Thai Quinoa Salad

Preparation Time: 10 minutes
Cooking Time: 0 minutes
Servings: 1-2
Ingredients:
Ingredients used for dressing:

- 1 tbsp. sesame seed
- 1 tsp. chopped garlic
- 1 tsp. lemon, fresh juice
- 3 tsp. apple cider vinegar
- 2 tsp. tamari, gluten-free.
- 1/4 cup of tahini (sesame butter)
- 1 pitted date
- 1/2 tsp. salt
- 1/2 tsp. toasted sesame oil

Salad ingredients:

- 1 cup of quinoa, steamed
- 1 big handful of arugula
- 1 tomato cut in pieces
- 1/4 of the red onion, diced

Directions:

1. Add the following to a small blender: 1/4 cup + 2 tbsp. Filtered water, the rest of the ingredients, and blend. Steam 1 cup of quinoa in a steamer or a rice pan, then set aside. Combine the quinoa, the arugula, the tomatoes sliced, the red onion diced on a serving plate or bowl, add the Thai dressing and serve with a spoon.

Nutrition:

- Calories: 100
- Carbohydrates: 12 g

38. Green Goddess Bowl and Avocado Cumin Dressing

Preparation Time: 10 minutes
Cooking Time: 0 minutes
Servings: 1-2
Ingredients:
Ingredients for the dressing of avocado cumin:

- 1 avocado
- 1 tbsp. cumin powder
- 2 limes, freshly squeezed
- 1 cup of filtered water
- 1/4 seconds. sea salt
- 1 tbsp. olive extra virgin olive oil
- Cayenne pepper dash
- Optional: 1/4 tsp. smoked pepper

Tahini lemon dressing ingredients:

- 1/4 cup of tahini (sesame butter)
- 1/2 cup of filtered water (more if you want thinner, less thick)
- 1/2 lemon, freshly squeezed
- 1 clove of minced garlic
- 3/4 tsp. sea salt (Celtic Gray, Himalayan, Redmond Real Salt)
- 1 tbsp. olive extra virgin olive oil
- Black pepper to taste

Salad ingredients:

- 3 cups of kale, chopped
- 1/2 cup of broccoli flowers, chopped
- 1/2 zucchini (make spiral noodles)
- 1/2 cup of kelp noodles, soaked and drained
- 1/3 cup of cherry tomatoes, halved.
- 2 tsp. hemp seeds

Directions:

1. Gently steam the kale and the broccoli (flash the steam for 4

minutes), set aside. Mix the zucchini noodles and kelp noodles and toss them with a generous portion of the smoked avocado cumin dressing. Add the cherry tomatoes and stir again. Place the steamed kale and broccoli and drizzle with the lemon tahini dressing. Top the kale and the broccoli with the noodles and tomatoes and sprinkle the whole dish with the hemp seeds.

Nutrition:

- Calories: 89
- Carbohydrates: 11g
- Fat: 1.2g
- Protein: 4g

39. Sweet and Savory Salad

Preparation Time: 10 minutes
Cooking Time: 0 minutes
Servings: 1-2
Ingredients:

- 1 big head of butter lettuce
- 1/2 of cucumber, sliced
- 1 pomegranate, seed or 1/3 cup of seed
- 1 avocado, 1 cubed
- 1/4 cup of shelled pistachio, chopped

Ingredients for dressing:

- 1/4 cup of apple cider vinegar
- 1/2 cup of olive oil
- 1 clove of garlic, minced

Directions:

1. Put the butter lettuce in a salad bowl. Add the remaining ingredients and toss with the salad dressing.

Nutrition:

- Calories: 68
- Carbohydrates: 8g
- Fat: 1.2g
- Protein: 2g

40. Kale Pesto's Pasta

Preparation Time: 10 minutes
Cooking Time: 0 minutes
Servings: 1-2
Ingredients:

- 1 bunch of kale
- 2 cups of fresh basil
- 1/4 cup of extra virgin olive oil
- 1/2 cup of walnuts
- 2 limes, freshly squeezed
- Sea salt and chili pepper
- 1 zucchini, noodle (spiralizer)
- Optional: garnish with chopped asparagus, spinach leaves, and tomato.

Directions:

1. The night before, soak the walnuts to improve absorption. Put all the recipe ingredients in a blender and blend until the consistency of the cream is reached. Add the zucchini noodles and enjoy.

Nutrition:

- Calories: 55
- Carbohydrates: 9 g
- Fat: 1.2g

41. Beet Salad with Basil Dressing

Preparation Time: 10 minutes
Cooking Time: 0 minutes
Servings: 4
Ingredients:

Ingredients for the dressing:

- ¼ cup blackberries
- ¼ cup extra-virgin olive oil
- Juice of 1 lemon
- 2 tablespoons minced fresh basil
- 1 teaspoon poppy seeds
- A pinch of sea salt

For the salad:

- 2 celery stalks, chopped
- 4 cooked beets, peeled and chopped
- 1 cup blackberries
- 4 cups spring mix

Directions:

1. To make the dressing, mash the blackberries in a bowl. Whisk in the oil, lemon juice, basil, poppy seeds, and sea salt.
2. To make the salad: Add the celery, beets, blackberries, and spring mix to the bowl with the dressing.
3. Combine and serve.

Nutrition:

- Calories: 192
- Fat: 15g
- Carbohydrates: 15g
- Protein: 2g

42. Basic Salad with Olive Oil Dressing

Preparation Time: 10 minutes
Cooking Time: 0 minute
Servings: 4
Ingredients:

- 1 cup coarsely chopped iceberg lettuce
- 1 cup coarsely chopped romaine lettuce
- 1 cup fresh baby spinach
- 1 large tomato, hulled and coarsely chopped
- 1 cup diced cucumber
- 2 tablespoons extra-virgin olive oil
- ¼ teaspoon of sea salt

Directions:

1. In a bowl, combine the spinach and lettuces. Add the tomato and cucumber.
2. Drizzle with oil and sprinkle with sea salt.
3. Mix and serve.

Nutrition:

- Calories: 77
- Fat: 4g
- Carbohydrates: 3g
- Protein: 1g

43. Spinach & Orange Salad with Oil Drizzle

Preparation Time: 10 minutes
Cooking Time: 0 minute
Servings: 4
Ingredients:

- 4 cups fresh baby spinach
- 1 blood orange, coarsely chopped
- ½ red onion, thinly sliced
- ½ shallot, finely chopped
- 2 tbsp. minced fennel fronds
- Juice of 1 lemon
- 1 tbsp. extra-virgin olive oil
- A pinch of sea salt

Directions:

1. In a bowl, toss together the spinach, orange, red onion, shallot, and fennel fronds.
2. Add the lemon juice, oil, and sea salt.
3. Mix and serve.

Nutrition:

- Calories: 79
- Fat: 2g
- Carbohydrates: 8g
- Protein: 1g

44. Fruit Salad with Coconut-Lime Dressing

Preparation Time: 5 minutes
Cooking Time: 0 minutes
Servings: 4
Ingredients:

Ingredients for the dressing:

- ¼ cup full-fat canned coconut milk
- 1 tbsp. raw honey
- Juice of ½ lime
- A pinch of sea salt

For the salad

- 2 bananas, thinly sliced
- 2 mandarin oranges, segmented
- ½ cup strawberries, thinly sliced
- ½ cup raspberries
- ½ cup blueberries

Directions:

1. To make the dressing: whisk all the dressing ingredients in a bowl.
2. To make the salad: Add the salad ingredients in a bowl and mix.
3. Drizzle with the dressing and serve.

Nutrition:

- Calories: 141
- Fat: 3g
- Carbohydrates: 30g
- Protein: 2g

45. Cranberry and Brussels Sprouts with Dressing

Preparation Time: 10 minutes
Cooking Time: 0 minute
Servings: 4
Ingredients:
Ingredients for the dressing:

- ⅓ cup extra-virgin olive oil
- 2 tbsp. apple cider vinegar
- 1 tbsp. pure maple syrup
- Juice of 1 orange
- ½ tbsp. dried rosemary
- 1 tbsp. scallion, whites only
- A pinch of sea salt

For the salad

- 1 bunch scallions, greens only, finely chopped
- 1 cup Brussels sprouts, stemmed, halved, and thinly sliced
- ½ cup fresh cranberries
- 4 cups fresh baby spinach

Directions:

1. To make the dressing: In a bowl, whisk the dressing ingredients.
2. To make the salad: Add the scallions, Brussels sprouts, cranberries, and spinach to the bowl with the dressing.
3. Combine and serve.

Nutrition:

- Calories: 267
- Fat: 18g
- Carbohydrates: 26g
- Protein: 2g

46. Parsnip, Carrot, and Kale Salad with Dressing

Preparation Time: 10 minutes
Cooking Time: 0 minutes
Servings: 4
Ingredients:
Ingredients for the dressing:

- ⅓ cup extra-virgin olive oil
- Juice of 1 lime
- 2 tbsp. minced fresh mint leaves
- 1 tsp. pure maple syrup
- A pinch of sea salt

For the salad:

- 1 bunch kale, chopped
- ½ parsnip, grated
- ½ carrot, grated
- 2 tbsp. sesame seeds

Directions:

1. To make the dressing, mix all the dressing ingredients in a bowl.
2. To make the salad, add the kale to the dressing and massage the dressing into the kale for 1 minute.
3. Add the parsnip, carrot, and sesame

seeds.
4. Combine and serve.

Nutrition:

- Calories: 214
- Fat: 2g
- Carbohydrates: 12g
- Protein: 2g

47. Tomato Toasts

Preparation Time: 5 minutes
Cooking Time: 5 minutes
Servings: 4
Ingredients:

- 4 slices of sprouted bread toasts
- 2 tomatoes, sliced
- 1 avocado, mashed
- 1 teaspoon olive oil
- 1 pinch of salt
- ¾ teaspoon ground black pepper

Directions:

1. Blend the olive oil, mashed avocado, salt, and ground black pepper.
2. When the mixture is homogenous – spread it over the sprouted bread.
3. Then place the sliced tomatoes over the toasts.
4. Enjoy!

Nutrition:

- Calories: 125
- Fat: 11.1g
- Carbohydrates: 7.0g
- Protein: 1.5g

48. Every day Salad

Preparation Time: 10 minutes
Cooking Time: 40 minutes
Servings: 6
Ingredients:

- 5 halved mushrooms
- 6 halved cherry (plum) tomatoes
- 6 rinsed lettuce leaves
- 10 olives
- ½ chopped cucumber
- Juice from ½ key lime
- 1 teaspoon olive oil
- Pure sea salt

Directions:

1. Tear rinsed lettuce leaves into medium pieces and put them in a medium salad bowl. Add mushrooms halves, chopped cucumber, olives, and cherry tomato halves into the bowl. Mix well. Pour olive and key lime juice over the salad. Add pure sea salt to taste. Mix it all till it is well combined.

Nutrition:

- Calories: 88
- Carbohydrates: 11g
- Fat: .5g
- Protein: .8g

49. Super-Seedy Salad with Tahini Dressing

Preparation Time: 10 minutes
Cooking Time: 0 minutes
Servings: 1-2
Ingredients:

- 1 slice stale sourdough, torn into chunks
- 50g mixed seeds
- 1 tsp. cumin seeds
- 1 tsp. coriander seeds
- 50g baby kale
- 75g long-stemmed broccoli, blanched for a few minutes then roughly chopped
- ½ red onion, thinly sliced
- 100g cherry tomatoes, halved
- ½ a small bunch flat-leaf parsley,

torn

DRESSING

- 100ml natural yogurt
- 1 tbsp. tahini
- 1 lemon, juiced

Directions:

1. Heat the oven to 200°C/fan 180°C/gas 6. Put the bread into a food processor and pulse into very rough breadcrumbs. Put into a bowl with the mixed seeds and spices, season, and spray well with oil. Tip onto a non-stick baking tray and roast for 15-20 minutes, stirring and tossing regularly, until deep golden brown.
2. Whisk together the dressing ingredients, some seasoning, and a splash of water in a large bowl. Tip the baby kale, broccoli, red onion, cherry tomatoes, and flat-leaf parsley into the dressing, and mix well. Divide between 2 plates and top with the crispy breadcrumbs and seeds.

Nutrition:

- Calories: 78
- Carbohydrates: 6 g
- Fat: 2g
- Protein: 1.5g

50. Sebi's Vegetable Salad

Preparation Time: 10 minutes
Cooking Time: 0 minutes
Servings: 1-2
Ingredients:

- 4 cups each of raw spinach and romaine lettuce
- 2 cups each of cherry tomatoes, sliced cucumber, chopped baby carrots and chopped red, orange and yellow bell pepper
- 1 cup each of chopped broccoli, sliced yellow squash, zucchini and cauliflower.

Directions:

1. Just wash all these vegetables. Mix in a large mixing bowl and top off with a non-fat or low-fat dressing of your choice.

Nutrition:

- Calories: 48
- Carbohydrates: 11g
- Protein: 3g

51. Greek Salad

Preparation Time: 10 minutes
Cooking Time: 0 minutes
Servings: 1-2
Ingredients:

- 1 Romaine head, torn in bits
- 1 cucumber sliced
- 1-pint cherry tomatoes, halved
- 1 green pepper, thinly sliced
- 1 onion sliced into rings
- 1 cup kalamata olives
- 1 ½ cups feta cheese, crumbled

For dressing combine:

- 1 cup olive oil
- 1/4 cup lemon juice
- 2 tsp. oregano
- Salt and pepper

Directions:

1. Layer ingredients on a plate. Drizzle dressing over salad.

Nutrition:

- Calories: 107
- Carbohydrates: 18g
- Fat: 1.2 g
- Protein: 1g

52. Sebi's Alkaline Spring Salad

Preparation Time: 10 minutes
Cooking Time: 0 minutes
Servings: 1-2

Eating seasonal fruits and vegetables is a fabulous way of taking care of yourself and the environment at the same time. This alkaline-electric salad is delicious and nutritious.

Ingredients:

- 4 cups seasonal approved greens of your choice
- 1 cup cherry tomatoes
- 1/4 cup walnuts
- 1/4 cup approved herbs of your choice

For the dressing:

- 3-4 key limes
- 1 tbsp. of homemade raw sesame
- Sea salt and cayenne pepper

Directions:

1. First, get the juice of the key limes. In a small bowl, whisk together the key lime juice with the homemade raw sesame "tahini" butter. Add sea salt and cayenne pepper, to taste.
2. Cut the cherry tomatoes in half.
3. In a large bowl, combine the greens, cherry tomatoes, and herbs. Pour the dressing on top and "massage" with your hands.
4. Let the greens soak up the dressing. Add more sea salt, cayenne pepper, and herbs on top if you wish. Enjoy!

Nutrition:

- Calories: 77
- Carbohydrates: 11g

Chapter 5: Main Dishes

53. Ginger-Maple Yam Casserole

Preparation Time: 10 minutes
Cooking Time: 40 minutes
Servings: 4
Ingredients:

- 2 yams, peeled and cut into ½-inch chunks
- ¼ cup fresh ginger, peeled and grated
- 2 tbsp. avocado oil
- 2 tbsp. pure maple syrup
- 4 tsp. cardamom
- A pinch of sea salt

Directions:

1. Preheat the oven to 375F.
2. In a casserole dish, combine the yams, ginger, oil, maple syrup, cardamom, and salt. Mix well.
3. Cover and bake for 40 minutes.
4. Serve.

Nutrition:

- Calories: 144
- Fat: 7g
- Carbohydrates: 20g
- Protein: 1g

54. Layered Cabbage Roll Casserole

Preparation Time: 10 minutes
Cooking Time: 40 minutes
Servings: 4
Ingredients:

- 1 cup quinoa
- ½ red onion, finely chopped
- 4 garlic cloves, minced
- 4 white mushrooms, finely chopped
- 1 (28-ounce) can diced tomatoes, drained
- 2 cups low-sodium vegetable stock
- ¼ cup minced fresh basil
- 8 green cabbage leaves, whole

Directions:

1. Preheat the oven to 350F.
2. In a casserole dish, combine 2 tbsp. red onion, ¼ cup quinoa, 1 minced garlic clove, and 1 chopped mushroom. Add ¼ can of tomatoes, ½ cup stock, and 1 tbsp. basil. Stir to mix.
3. Top with 2 cabbage leaves. Repeat steps 2 and 3 until all of the ingredients are used up.
4. Cover and bake for 40 minutes.
5. Rest for 10 minutes and serve.

Nutrition:

- Calories: 261
- Fat: 2g
- Carbohydrates: 51g
- Protein: 12g

55. Vegetarian Pie

Preparation Time: 20 minutes
Cooking Time: 1 hour 20 minutes
Servings: 8
Ingredients:

Ingredients for topping:

- 5 cups of water
- 1¼ cups yellow cornmeal

For filing:

- 1 tbsp. extra-virgin olive oil
- 1 large onion, chopped
- 1 medium red bell pepper, seeded and chopped
- 2 garlic cloves, minced
- 1 tsp. dried oregano, crushed

- 2 tsp. chili powder
- 2 cups fresh tomatoes, chopped
- 2½ cups cooked pinto beans
- 2 cups boiled corn kernels

Directions:

1. Preheat the oven to 375 F. Lightly grease a shallow baking dish.
2. In a pan, add the water over medium-high heat and bring to a boil.
3. Slowly, add the cornmeal, stirring continuously.
4. Reduce the heat to low and cook covered for about 20 minutes, stirring occasionally.
5. Meanwhile, prepare the filling. In a large skillet, heat the oil over medium heat and sauté the onion and bell pepper for about 3-4 minutes.
6. Add the garlic, oregano, and spices and sauté for about 1 minute
7. Add the remaining ingredients and stir to combine.
8. Reduce the heat to low and simmer for about 10-15 minutes, stirring occasionally.
9. Remove from the heat.
10. Place half of the Cooked cornmeal into the Prepared baking dish evenly.
11. Place the filling mixture over the cornmeal evenly.
12. Place the remaining cornmeal over the filling mixture evenly.
13. Bake for 45-50 minutes or until the top becomes golden brown.
14. Remove the pie from the oven and set it aside for about 5 minutes before serving.

Nutrition:

- Calories: 350
- Fat: 3.9g
- Carbohydrates: 58.2g
- Protein: 16.8g

56. Ginger-Sesame Quinoa with Vegetables

Preparation Time: 10 minutes
Cooking Time: 30 minutes
Servings: 4
Ingredients:

- 1 cup quinoa
- 2 cups low-sodium vegetable stock
- 1 tbsp. tahini
- 4 tsp. fresh ginger, peeled and minced
- A pinch of sea salt, plus more for seasoning
- 2 carrots, finely chopped
- 1 red bell pepper, finely chopped
- 1 cup snow peas, stringed and halved
- 2 tsp. sesame seeds
- Sesame oil, for garnish

Directions:

1. Preheat the oven to 325F.
2. In a casserole dish, combine the stock, quinoa, tahini, ginger, and salt. Mix.
3. Add in the pepper, carrots, and snow peas. Mix well.
4. Cover and bake for 30 minutes.
5. Top with sesame seeds and a drizzle of sesame oil.
6. Adjust seasoning with salt and serve.

Nutrition:

- Calories: 261
- Fat: 3g
- Carbohydrates: 46g
- Protein: 10g

57. Butternut Squash, Apple Casserole with Drizzle

Preparation Time: 10 minutes
Cooking Time: 30 minutes

Servings: 4

Ingredients:

- 1 butternut squash, peeled, seeded, and cut into ½-inch chunks
- 2 Granny Smith apples, cored and cut into ½-inch chunks
- 1 white onion, cut into ½-inch chunks
- 4 garlic cloves, coarsely chopped
- ½ tbsp. avocado oil
- ½ tbsp. pure maple syrup
- 2 tsp. ground cinnamon
- ½ tsp. chili powder
- A pinch of sea salt
- A pinch of freshly ground black pepper

Directions:

1. Preheat the oven to 375F.
2. In a large casserole dish, combine the apples, squash, onion, garlic, oil, syrup, cinnamon, chili powder, salt, and pepper. Mix well.
3. Cover and bake for 30 minutes.
4. Serve.

Nutrition:

- Calories: 123
- Fat: 2g
- Carbohydrates: 28g
- Protein: 2g

58. Mango, Quinoa, and Black Bean Casserole with Sauce

Preparation Time: 10 minutes

Cooking Time: 25 minutes

Servings: 4

Ingredients:

- 2 cups full-fat canned coconut milk
- 1 cup low-sodium vegetable stock
- 1 cup quinoa
- 2 cups black beans, drained and rinsed
- 1 mango, finely chopped
- ¼ cup minced fresh mint
- A pinch of sea salt, for seasoning

Directions:

1. Preheat the oven to 425F.
2. In a casserole dish, combine the stock, milk, and quinoa.
3. Cover and bake for 25 minutes.
4. Remove the dish from the oven. Mix in the beans, mango, and fresh mint.
5. Season with salt and serve.

Nutrition:

- Calories: 573
- Fat: 23g
- Carbohydrates: 75g
- Protein: 15g

59. Pepper and Onion Masala

Preparation Time: 10 minutes

Cooking Time: 30 minutes

Servings: 2

Ingredients:

- 1 cup of brown rice
- Boiling filtered water, for rinsing
- 2 tablespoons coconut oil
- 1 teaspoon cumin seeds
- ¼ teaspoon asafoetida
- ½ teaspoon ground turmeric
- 1 onion, rinsed and chopped
- 2 green chiles, rinsed and chopped
- 2 garlic cloves, chopped
- 1 (1-inch) piece fresh ginger, peeled and grated
- 3 tablespoons tomato paste
- 1 teaspoon chili powder
- Himalayan pink salt
- 1 bell pepper, any color, rinsed and chopped
- 2 tablespoons of filtered water

Directions:

1. In a minor saucepan over average-low heat, associate the brown rice with enough boiling water to cover, and simmer for 25 to 30 minutes, until cooked. Drain and rinse with boiling filtered water.
2. Meanwhile, in a small non-stick skillet over medium heat, heat the coconut oil. Add the cumin seeds, asafoetida, and turmeric. Fry for 3 minutes, until golden.
3. Add the onion, green chiles, garlic, and ginger. Sauté for 5 minutes, until the onion is soft.
4. Stir in the tomato paste and chili powder, and season with salt. Mix well.
5. Add the bell pepper and water, and cook for 5 minutes.
6. Serve the rice with the hot masala.

Nutrition:

- Calories: 520
- Total fat: 8g
- Total carbohydrates: 81g
- Fiber: 6g
- Sugar: 4g
- Protein: 4g

60. Red Thai Vegetable Curry

Preparation Time: 10 minutes
Cooking Time: 15 minutes
Servings: 4
Ingredients:

- 2 cups vegetable stock
- 1 sweet potato, rinsed and chopped
- 1 head broccoli, rinsed and chopped
- 1 eggplant, rinsed and chopped
- 1 zucchini, rinsed and chopped
- 1 red bell pepper, rinsed and chopped
- 1½ cups canned, full-fat coconut milk
- 1 tablespoon red Thai curry paste
- 2 kaffir lime leaves
- 1 (1-inch) piece fresh ginger, peeled and grated
- Himalayan pink salt
- Freshly ground black pepper
- 2 tablespoons coconut aminos
- Juice of 1 lime

Directions:

1. In a large pot over high heat, bring the vegetable stock to a boil. Add the sweet potato, broccoli, eggplant, zucchini, red bell pepper, coconut milk, curry paste, lime leaves, and ginger. Reduce the heat to low and cook for 10 minutes, stirring frequently. Taste and season with salt and pepper. Simmer for 5 minutes more.
2. Remove the pot from the heat, stir in the coconut aminos and lime juice, and serve.

Nutrition:

- Calories: 300
- Total fat: 19g
- Total carbohydrates: 23g
- Fiber: 9g
- Sugar: 11g
- Protein: 7g

61. Thick Alkaline Minestrone

Preparation Time: 10 minutes
Cooking Time: 15 minutes
Servings: 2
Ingredients:

- 1 tablespoon coconut oil
- ¼ onion, rinsed and diced
- 2 garlic cloves, minced
- ½ cup sweet potato, scrubbed and cubed

- ½ cup zucchini, rinsed and cubed
- ½ cup eggplant, rinsed and cubed
- ½ cup carrot, rinsed and diced
- ½ cup canned beans, such as white, navy, or kidney beans, rinsed and drained
- 1 cup tomato juice
- ½ cup vegetable stock
- Handful fresh basil leaves, rinsed
- Himalayan pink salt
- Freshly ground black pepper

Directions:

1. In a large pot over medium-high heat, heat the coconut oil. Add the onion, garlic, sweet potato, zucchini, eggplant, and carrot. Sauté for 3 minutes.
2. Stir in the beans, tomato juice, and vegetable stock. Bring to a boil. Reduce the heat to simmer and cook for 10 minutes.
3. Stir in the basil, season with salt and pepper, and serve.

Nutrition:

- Calories: 168
- Total fat: 7g
- Total carbohydrates: 25g
- Fiber: 6g
- Sugar: 11g
- Protein: 4g

62. Pesto Soba Noodles

Preparation Time: 5 minutes
Cooking Time: 15 minutes
Servings: 2
Ingredients:

- 3 tablespoons extra-virgin olive oil
- 1 bunch fresh basil leaves, rinsed
- 1 bunch fresh parsley, rinsed
- 1 bunch fresh cilantro, rinsed
- 3½ ounces soba buckwheat noodles, cooked according to package directions
- Himalayan pink salt
- Freshly ground black pepper

Directions:

1. In a blender, combine the olive oil, basil, parsley, and cilantro. Blend until smooth.
2. In a large bowl, combine the cooked noodles and sauce. Toss to coat, season with salt and pepper, and serve.

Nutrition:

- Calories: 355
- Total fat: 21g
- Total carbohydrates: 36g
- Fiber: 1g
- Sugar: 0g
- Protein: 9g

63. Quinoa Burrito Bowl

Preparation Time: 10 minutes
Cooking Time: 10 minutes
Servings: 4
Ingredients:

- 1 cup quinoa, rinsed well
- Boiling filtered water
- 1 can of black beans, washed and rinsed
- 4 scallions, white parts only, rinsed and sliced
- 4 garlic cloves, minced
- 1 teaspoon ground cumin
- 1 teaspoon red pepper flakes
- Juice of 2 limes
- 2 avocados, peeled, pitted, and sliced
- Handful fresh cilantro, rinsed and chopped

Directions:

1. In a small saucepan over medium heat, combine the quinoa with enough boiling water to shield and then simmer for 8 to 10 minutes, until the water has absorbed. Drain, rinse and set aside.
2. Meanwhile, in another small saucepan over low heat, stir together the black beans, scallions, garlic, cumin, red pepper flakes, and lime juice. Simmer for 10 minutes to warm.
3. In a large bowl, stir collected the quinoa and warmed beans. Top with the avocado and cilantro and serve.

Nutrition:

- Calories: 420
- Total fat: 9g
- Carbohydrates: 70g
- Fiber: 18g
- Sugar: 2g
- Protein: 10g

64. Millet Pilaf

Preparation Time: 10 minutes
Cooking Time: 15 minutes
Servings: 4
Ingredients:

- 1 cup millet
- 2 tomatoes, rinsed, seeded, and chopped
- 1¾ cups of filtered water
- 2 tablespoons extra-virgin olive oil
- ¼ cup chopped dried apricot
- Zest of 1 lemon
- Juice of 1 lemon
- ½ cup fresh parsley, rinsed and chopped
- Himalayan pink salt
- Freshly ground black pepper

Directions:

1. In an electric pressure cooker, combine the millet, tomatoes, and water. Lock the lid into place, select manual and high pressure, and cook for 7 minutes.
2. When the beep sounds, quick release the pressure by pressing Cancel and twisting the steam valve to the Venting position. Carefully remove the lid.
3. Stir in the olive oil, apricot, lemon zest, lemon juice, and parsley. Taste, season with salt and pepper, and serve.

Nutrition:

- Calories: 270
- Total fat: 8g
- Total carbohydrates: 42g
- Fiber: 5g
- Sugar: 3g
- Protein: 6g

65. Basil and Olive Pizza

Preparation Time: 10 minutes
Cooking Time: 30 minutes
Servings: 4
Ingredients:

FOR THE PIZZA SAUCE

- 1 (15-ounce) can tomatoes
- 1 tablespoon extra-virgin olive oil
- ½ cup fresh basil leaves, rinsed
- 2 garlic cloves, chopped
- 1 teaspoon onion powder
- ¼ teaspoon dried oregano
- ¼ teaspoon dried sage
- ¼ teaspoon dried rosemary
- ¼ teaspoon red chili flakes (optional)
- 1 teaspoon Himalayan pink salt
- Pinch freshly ground black pepper

FOR THE PIZZAS

- 4 spelt flour pita slices of bread
- 4 ounces' vegan mozzarella, shredded
- 1 cup mixed veggies of your choice (tomatoes, eggplant, onion, green pepper, mushroom, etc.), rinsed and finely sliced
- ⅔ cup pitted olives, chopped
- 1 tablespoon extra-virgin olive oil
- 5 fresh basil leaves, rinsed and torn

Directions:

TO MAKE THE PIZZA SAUCE

1. In a blender, blend the tomatoes, olive oil, basil, garlic, onion powder, oregano, sage, rosemary, chili flakes, salt, and pepper on low until the basil and garlic are in very small pieces.
2. Transfer to a pot over middle heat and simmer for about 20 minutes, until the sauce reduces slightly and thickens.

TO MAKE THE PIZZAS

1. Preheat the oven to 500°F. Line a baking sheet with parchment paper and set aside.
2. Spread the pizza sauce evenly over the pitas. Top with the vegan mozzarella and scatter the sliced veggies and olives on top.
3. Bake for 8 minutes, or until golden on top.
4. Drizzle the pizzas with the olive oil and scatter the basil leaves over them. Freeze leftovers in an airtight container for up to three weeks.

Nutrition:

- Calories: 400
- Total fat: 10g
- Total carbohydrates: 64g
- Fiber: 5g
- Sugar: 2g
- Protein: 10g

66. Black Bean Chili

Preparation Time: 15 minutes
Cooking Time: 20 minutes
Servings: 4
Ingredients:

- 1 tablespoon coconut oil
- 1 small onion, rinsed and diced
- 6 mushrooms, cleaned and sliced
- 2 tablespoons ground coriander
- 2 tablespoons paprika
- 2 tablespoons ground cumin
- 1 tablespoon ground cinnamon
- 1 tablespoon ground nutmeg
- 1 tablespoon chili powder
- 1 (15-ounce) can tomatoes
- 1 can of black beans, washed and rinsed
- 1 (15.5-ounce) can kidney beans, rinsed and drained
- 5 cherry tomatoes, rinsed
- 2 tablespoons tomato purée
- 1 tablespoon raw honey or agave nectar
- ½ cup red wine or grape juice
- 3 squares dark chocolate, or 1 heaping tablespoon cocoa powder
- 7 ounces uncooked brown rice
- 4 tablespoons coconut yogurt, for serving (optional)
- 4 fresh cilantro sprigs, for serving (optional)

Directions:

1. In a great pan over average heat, heat the coconut oil. Include the onion and mushrooms, and sauté for 5 minutes. Stir in the coriander, paprika, cumin, cinnamon, nutmeg, and chili powder.
2. Add the canned tomatoes with their

juices, black beans, kidney beans, cherry tomatoes, and tomato purée. Mix to combine and carry to a simmer. Cook for 5 minutes.
3. Stir in the honey, wine, and chocolate. Turn the heat to little and simmer for 10 minutes.
4. While the chili cooks, cook the rice according to the package directions. Rinse and drain.
5. Serve the chili above the rice, garnished with yogurt (if using), and cilantro (if using).

Nutrition:

- Calories: 580g
- Total fat: 5g
- Total carbohydrates: 102g
- Fiber: 18g
- Sugar: 14g
- Protein: 19g

67. Mixed Lentils

Preparation Time: 15 minutes
Cooking Time: 30 minutes
Servings: 4
Ingredients:

- 2 tablespoons coconut oil
- 1 onion, rinsed and diced
- 2 carrots, rinsed and diced
- 2 celery stalks, rinsed and diced
- 1 sweet potato, rinsed and diced
- 1 cup dried red lentils
- 1 cup dried puy lentils
- 5 cups vegetable stock
- Himalayan pink salt
- Freshly ground black pepper

Directions:

1. In a large pot over medium heat, heat the coconut oil. Include the onion and fry for 3 minutes, or until it has softened.
2. Supplement the carrots, celery, and sweet potato, and cook for 2 minutes.
3. Add the red and puy lentils and vegetable stock. Carry to a boil and lower the heat to simmer. Cook this for 25 minutes, or until the lentils are soft. Season with salt and pepper and serve.

Nutrition:

- Calories: 330
- Total fat: 10g
- Total carbohydrates: 49g
- Fiber: 20g
- Sugar: 8g
- Protein: 17g

68. Zucchini-Broccoli Stir-Fry

Preparation Time: 15 minutes
Cooking Time: 15 minutes
Servings: 4
Ingredients:

- 2 tablespoons coconut oil
- 2 tablespoons sesame oil
- 1 (2-inch) piece fresh ginger, peeled and finely chopped
- 4 garlic cloves, minced
- 2 onions, rinsed and chopped
- 1 head broccoli, rinsed and broken into florets
- 1 zucchini, rinsed and cut into long, fettuccine-like strips
- 3 scallions, white parts only, rinsed and chopped
- 1 tablespoon fresh basil leaves, rinsed and chopped
- 1-ounce coconut aminos

Directions:

1. In a wok or large skillet over medium heat, heat the coconut and sesame oils. Mix the ginger and garlic and sauté for 5 minutes, until fragrant.

2. Add the onion and broccoli, and cook for 3 minutes, until the onion softens slightly.
3. Add the zucchini, scallions, and basil. Stir to combine and heat for 4 minutes, until the vegetables are tender.
4. Remove the wok from the heat, sprinkle in the coconut aminos, and serve.

Nutrition:

- Calories: 180
- Total fat: 14g
- Total carbohydrates: 13g
- Fiber: 3g
- Sugar: 4g
- Protein: 3g

69. Tomato Spelt Pasta

Preparation Time: 15 minutes
Cooking Time: 20 minutes
Servings: 4
Ingredients:

- 3 tablespoons extra-virgin olive oil
- 2 garlic cloves, crushed
- 1 onion, rinsed and diced
- 1 eggplant, rinsed and diced
- 2 zucchinis, rinsed and diced
- 3 tomatoes, rinsed and diced
- ⅔ cup sun-dried tomatoes
- 2 teaspoons dried basil
- 1 teaspoon dried oregano
- 1 cup vegetable stock
- 1 tablespoon red wine vinegar
- Himalayan pink salt
- Freshly ground black pepper
- 7 ounces spelt pasta
- Boiling filtered water

Directions:

1. In a great pan over average heat, heat the olive oil. Add the garlic, onion, and eggplant, and sauté for 8 minutes.
2. Add the zucchini, tomatoes, sun-dried tomatoes, basil, and oregano. Cook for 8 minutes, stirring.
3. Stir in the vegetable stock and vinegar, and season with salt and pepper. Let simmer for a few minutes.
4. Meanwhile, in a separate, saucepan over medium heat, combine the pasta with enough boiling water to cover and cook for about 10 minutes, until soft. Drain.
5. Serve the pasta with the sauce.

Nutrition:

- Calories: 460
- Total fat: 12g
- Total carbohydrates: 75g
- Fiber: 10g
- Sugar: 11g
- Protein: 17g

70. Green Tomatoes Crisps

Preparation Time: 14 minutes
Cooking Time: 16 minutes
Servings: 3
Ingredients:

- ¼ cup coconut flour
- A pinch of salt
- A pinch of pepper
- 4 green tomatoes
- 1 cup applesauce
- ½ cup almond flour
- ¼ cup olive oil

Directions:

1. First is to mix the coconut flour, salt, and pepper in a bowl. Mix the tomatoes. Toss until well coated.
2. In another bowl, pour applesauce.

Add almond flour. Mix until well combined.

3. Heat the oil. Dip the tomatoes into the applesauce mixture and the almond mixture. Fry tomatoes in batches until golden brown. Serve.

Nutrition:

- Calories 113
- Total Fat 4.2 g
- Saturated Fat 0.8 g
- Cholesterol 0 mg
- Sodium 861 mg
- Total Carbs 22.5 g
- Fiber 6.3 g
- Sugar 2.3 g
- Protein 9.2 g

71. Fruit Salad in Cider

Preparation Time: 11 minutes
Cooking Time: 16 minutes
Servings: 3
Ingredients:

For the salad:

- 1 piece, small apple, cubed
- 1 piece, small apricot, cubed
- 1/4 piece, small grapefruit pulp, shredded into bite-sized pieces
- 1/4 cup, loosely packed jicama, cubed

For cider sauce:

- 2 tbsp. apple cider vinegar, warmed in the microwave oven
- A dash of cinnamon powder

Directions:

1. Combine apple cider vinegar and cinnamon powder in a small bowl. Mix well.
2. Place salad ingredients in a large bowl; pour in cider sauce. Toss well to combine; spoon equal portions into plates. Serve immediately.

Nutrition:

- Calories 123
- Total Fat 14.2 g
- Saturated Fat 0.7 g
- Cholesterol 0 mg
- Sodium 661 mg
- Total Carbs 22.5 g
- Fiber 6.3 g
- Sugar 2.9 g
- Protein 9.2 g

72. Roasted Vegetables

Preparation Time: 14 minutes
Cooking Time: 17 minutes
Servings: 3
Ingredients:

- 4 Tbsp. olive oil, reserve some for greasing
- 2 heads, large garlic, tops sliced off
- 2 large eggplants/aubergine, tops removed, cubed
- 2 large shallots, peeled, quartered
- 1 large carrot, peeled, cubed
- 1 large parsnip, peeled, cubed
- 1 small green bell pepper, deseeded, ribbed, cubed
- 1 small red bell pepper, deseeded, ribbed, cubed
- 1/2 pound Brussels sprouts, halved, do not remove cores
- 1 sprig, large thyme, leaves picked
- Sea salt, coarse-grained

For garnish:

- 1 large lemon, halved, 1/2 squeezed, 1/2 sliced into smaller wedges
- 1/8 cup fennel bulb, minced

Directions:

1. Preheat the oven to 425°F or 220°C for at least 5 minutes before using.
2. Line deep roasting pan with

aluminium foil; lightly grease with oil. Tumble in bell peppers, Brussels sprouts, carrots, eggplants, garlic, parsnips, rosemary leaves, shallots, and thyme. Add a pinch of sea salt; drizzle in remaining oil and lemon juice. Toss well to combine.

3. Cover roasting pan with a sheet of aluminium foil. Place this on the middle rack of the oven. Bake for 20 to 30 minutes. Remove aluminium foil. Roast, for another 5 to 10 minutes, or until some vegetables brown at the edges. Remove roasting pan from the oven. Cool slightly before ladling equal portions into plates.
4. Garnish with fennel and a wedge of lemon. Squeeze lemon juice on top of the dish before eating.

Nutrition:

- Calories 163
- Total Fat 4.2 g
- Saturated Fat 0.8 g
- Cholesterol 0 mg
- Sodium 861 mg
- Total Carbs 22.5 g
- Fiber 6.3 g
- Sugar 2.3 g
- Protein 9.2 g

73. Sweet and Sour Onions

Preparation Time: 10 minutes
Cooking Time: 11 minutes
Servings: 4
Ingredients:

- 4 large onions, halved
- 2 garlic cloves, crushed
- 3 cups vegetable stock
- 1 ½ tablespoon balsamic vinegar
- ½ teaspoon Dijon mustard
- 1 tablespoon sugar

Directions:

1. Combine onions and garlic in a pan. Fry for 3 minutes, or till softened.
2. Pour stock, vinegar, Dijon mustard, and sugar. Bring to a boil.
3. Reduce heat. Cover and let the combination simmer for 10 minutes.
4. Get rid of from heat. Continue stirring until the liquid is reduced and the onions are brown. Serve.

Nutrition:

- Calories 203
- Total Fat 41.2 g
- Saturated Fat 0.8 g
- Cholesterol 0 mg
- Sodium 861 mg
- Total Carbs 29.5 g
- Fiber 16.3 g
- Sugar 29.3 g
- Protein 19.2 g

74. Sautéed Apples and Onions

Preparation Time: 14 minutes
Cooking Time: 16 minutes
Servings: 3
Ingredients:

- 2 cups dry cider
- 1 large onion, halved
- 2 cups vegetable stock
- 4 apples, sliced into wedges
- A pinch of salt
- A pinch of pepper

Directions:

1. Combine cider and onion in a saucepan. Bring to a boil until the onions are cooked and liquid is almost gone.
2. Pour the stock and the apples. Season with salt and pepper. Stir occasionally. Cook for about 10

minutes or until the apples are tender but not mushy. Serve.

Nutrition:

- Calories 343
- Total Fat 51.2 g
- Saturated Fat 0.8 g
- Cholesterol 0 mg
- Sodium 861 mg
- Total Carbs 22.5 g
- Fiber 6.3 g
- Sugar 2.3 g
- Protein 9.2 g

75. Zucchini Noodles with Portabella Mushrooms

Preparation Time: 14 minutes
Cooking Time: 16 minutes
Servings: 3
Ingredients:

- 1 zucchini, processed into spaghetti-like noodles
- 3 garlic cloves, minced
- 2 white onions, thinly sliced
- 1 thumb-sized ginger, julienned
- 1 lb. chicken thighs
- 1 lb. portabella mushrooms, sliced into thick slivers
- 2 cups chicken stock
- 3 cups of water
- A pinch of sea salt, add more if needed
- A pinch of black pepper, add more if needed
- 2 tsp. sesame oil
- 4 tbsp. coconut oil, divided
- ¼ cup fresh chives, minced, for garnish

Directions:

1. Pour 2 tablespoons of coconut oil into a large saucepan. Fry mushroom slivers in batches for 5 minutes or until seared brown. Set aside. Transfer these to a plate.
2. Sauté the onion, garlic, and ginger for 3 minutes or until tender. Add in chicken thighs, cooked mushrooms, chicken stock, water, salt, and pepper stir mixture well. Bring to a boil.
3. Decrease gradually the heat and allow simmering for 20 minutes or until the chicken is forking tender. Tip in sesame oil.
4. Serve by placing an equal amount of zucchini noodles into bowls. Ladle soup and garnish with chives.

Nutrition:

- Calories 163
- Total Fat 4.2 g
- Saturated Fat 0.8 g
- Cholesterol 0 mg
- Sodium 861 mg
- Total Carbs 22.5 g
- Fiber 6.3 g
- Sugar 2.3 g
- Protein 9.2 g

76. Grilled Tempeh with Pineapple

Preparation Time: 12 minutes
Cooking Time: 16 minutes
Servings: 3
Ingredients:

- 10 oz. tempeh, sliced
- 1 red bell pepper, quartered
- 1/4 pineapple, sliced into rings
- 6 oz. green beans
- 1 tbsp. coconut aminos
- 2 1/2 tbsp. orange juice, freshly squeeze
- 1 1/2 tbsp. lemon juice, freshly

squeezed
- 1 tbsp. extra virgin olive oil
- 1/4 cup hoisin sauce

Directions:

1. Blend the olive oil, orange and lemon juices, coconut aminos or soy sauce, and hoisin sauce in a bowl. Add the diced tempeh and set aside.
2. Heat up the grill or place a grill pan over medium-high flame. Once hot, lift the marinated tempeh from the bowl with a pair of tongs and transfer them to the grill or pan.
3. Grill for 2 to 3 minutes, or until browned all over.
4. Grill the sliced pineapples alongside the tempeh, then transfer them directly onto the serving platter.
5. Place the grilled tempeh beside the grilled pineapple and cover with aluminium foil to keep warm.
6. Meanwhile, place the green beans and bell peppers in a bowl and add just enough of the marinade to coat.
7. Prepare the grill pan and add the vegetables. Grill until fork tender and slightly charred.
8. Transfer the grilled vegetables to the serving platter and arrange artfully with the tempeh and pineapple. Serve at once.

Nutrition:

- Calories 163
- Total Fat 4.2 g
- Saturated Fat 0.8 g
- Cholesterol 0 mg
- Sodium 861 mg
- Total Carbs 22.5 g
- Fiber 6.3 g
- Sugar 2.3 g
- Protein 9.2 g

77. Courgettes in Cider Sauce

Preparation Time: 13 minutes
Cooking Time: 17 minutes
Servings: 3
Ingredients:

- 2 cups baby courgettes
- 3 tablespoons vegetable stock
- 2 tablespoons apple cider vinegar
- 1 tablespoon light brown sugar
- 4 spring onions, finely sliced
- 1 piece of fresh ginger root, grated
- 1 teaspoon of corn flour
- 2 teaspoons of water

Directions:

- Bring a pan with salted water to a boil. Add courgettes. Bring to a boil for 5 minutes.
- Meanwhile, in a pan, combine vegetable stock, apple cider vinegar, brown sugar, onions, ginger root, lemon juice and rind, and orange juice and rind. Take to a boil. Lower the heat and allow simmering for 3 minutes.
- Mix the corn flour with water. Stir well. Pour into the sauce. Continue stirring until the sauce thickens.
- Drain courgettes. Transfer to the serving dish. Spoon over the sauce. Toss to coat courgettes. Serve.

Nutrition:

- Calories 173
- Total Fat 9.2 g
- Saturated Fat 0.8 g
- Cholesterol 0 mg
- Sodium 861 mg
- Total Carbs 22.5 g
- Fiber 6.3 g
- Sugar 2.3 g
- Protein 9.2 g

78. Baked Mixed Mushrooms

Preparation Time: 8 minutes
Cooking Time: 20 minutes
Servings: 3
Ingredients:

- 2 cups mixed wild mushrooms
- 1 cup chestnut mushrooms
- 2 cups dried porcini
- 2 shallots
- 4 garlic cloves
- 3 cups raw pecans
- ½ bunch fresh thyme
- 1 bunch flat-leaf parsley
- 2 tablespoons olive oil
- 2 fresh bay leaves
- 1 ½ cups stale bread

Directions:

1. Remove skin and finely chop garlic and shallots. Roughly chop the wild mushrooms and chestnut mushrooms. Pick the leaves of the thyme and tear the bread into small pieces. Put inside the pressure cooker.
2. Place the pecans and roughly chop the nuts. Pick the parsley leaves and roughly chop.
3. Place the porcini in a bowl then add 300ml of boiling water. Set aside until needed.
4. Heat oil in the pressure cooker. Add the garlic and shallots. Cook for 3 minutes while stirring occasionally.
5. Drain porcini and reserve the liquid. Add the porcini into the pressure cooker together with the wild mushrooms and chestnut mushrooms. Add the bay leaves and thyme.
6. Position the lid and lock in place. Put to high heat and bring to high pressure. Adjust heat to stabilize. Cook for 10 minutes. Adjust taste if necessary.
7. Transfer the mushroom mixture into a bowl and set aside to cool completely.
8. Once the mushrooms are completely cool, add the bread, pecans, a pinch of black pepper and sea salt, and half of the reserved liquid into the bowl. Mix well. Add more reserved liquid if the mixture seems dry.
9. Add more than half of the parsley into the bowl and stir. Transfer the mixture into a 20cm x 25cm lightly greased baking dish and cover with tin foil.
10. Bake in the oven for 35 minutes. Then, get rid of the foil and cook for another 10 minutes. Once done, sprinkle the remaining parsley on top and serve with bread or crackers. Serve.

Nutrition:

- Calories 343
- Total Fat 4.2 g
- Saturated Fat 0.8 g
- Cholesterol 0 mg
- Sodium 861 mg
- Total Carbs 22.5 g
- Fiber 6.3 g
- Sugar 2.3 g
- Protein 9.2 g

79. Spiced Okra

Preparation Time: 14 minutes
Cooking Time: 16 minutes
Servings: 3
Ingredients:

- 2 cups okra
- ¼ teaspoon stevia

- 1 teaspoon chilli powder
- ½ teaspoon ground turmeric
- 1 tablespoon ground coriander
- 2 tablespoons fresh coriander, chopped
- 1 tablespoon ground cumin
- ¼ teaspoon salt
- 1 tablespoon desiccated coconut
- 3 tablespoons vegetable oil
- ½ teaspoon black mustard seeds
- ½ teaspoon cumin seeds
- Fresh tomatoes, to garnish

Directions:

1. Trim the okra. Wash and dry.
2. Combine stevia, chilli powder, turmeric, ground coriander, fresh coriander, cumin, salt, and desiccated coconut in a bowl.
3. Heat the oil in a pan. Cook mustard and cumin seeds for 3 minutes. Stir continuously. Add okra. Tip in the spice mixture. Cook on low heat for 8 minutes.
4. Transfer to a serving dish. Garnish with fresh tomatoes.

Nutrition:

- Calories 163
- Total Fat 4.2 g
- Saturated Fat 0.8 g
- Cholesterol 0 mg
- Sodium 861 mg
- Total Carbs 22.5 g
- Fiber 6.3 g
- Sugar 2.3 g
- Protein 9.2 g

Chapter 6: Sauces

80. Alkaline Salsa Mexicana

Preparation Time: 14 minutes
Cooking Time: 16 minutes
Servings: 3
Ingredients:

- Cayenne pepper, one (1) pinch
- Spring onions, two (2)
- Tomatoes (big), three (3)
- Cilantro (a handful)
- Juice of lime, one (1)
- Organic or sea salt (one pinch)
- Chilies (green), two (2)
- Garlic, two (2) cloves

Directions:

1. Chop garlic cloves in tiny pieces, cut the chilies in small pieces, cut the onions in rings, and put the tomatoes in small cubes.
2. There are two ways you can about it, depend on how you prefer your salsa (either smooth or chunky).
3. For a smooth salsa; add all the ingredients in a mixing pan and mix well.
4. Empty the mix in a food processor and blast for a few seconds.
5. Add salt and pepper to taste.
6. Serve.
7. However, for a chunky salsa; add all ingredients together in a mixing bowl and mix properly.
8. Add salt and pepper to taste.
9. Serve.

Nutrition:

- Calories: 5
- Carbohydrates: 1g

81. Tofu Salad Dressing

Preparation Time: 14 minutes
Cooking Time: 16 minutes
Servings: 3
Ingredients:

- Stevia powder, one (1) teaspoon
- Tofu, 100g
- Alkaline water, Five (5) tablespoons
- Random spices and herbs of your choice
- Sea salt, ½ teaspoon

Directions:

1. Include all elements in a food processor and process until it is fine to consistency.
2. Enjoy it with salad.

Nutrition:

- Calories: 80
- Carbohydrates: 1g
- Fat: 9g
- Protein: 1g

82. Millet Spread

Preparation Time: 14 minutes
Cooking Time: 16 minutes
Servings: 3
Ingredients:

- Pepper, one (1) pinch
- White onion (big), one (1)
- Millet, one (1) cup
- Any garden herb of your choice, one (1) teaspoon
- Virgin olive oil (cold-pressed extra), one (1) tablespoon
- Alkaline water, two (2) cups
- Organic/sea salt, one (1) pinch
- Yeast-free vegetable stock, one (1) teaspoon

Directions:

1. Get a small pot over medium heat, add water, the vegetable stock, and millet and boil for ten minutes, and put the pot aside for some minutes.
2. In a different pan, add oil and stir fry the roughly chopped onion.
3. Once that is done, add the stir-fried onion to the millet.
4. Mix properly, then add salt and pepper to taste.
5. Place it in a mixer and blend for 40 seconds.
6. Serve.

Nutrition:

- Calories: 25
- Carbohydrates: 5 g

83. Alkaline Eggplant Dip

Preparation Time: 14 minutes
Cooking Time: 16 minutes
Servings: 3
Ingredients:

- Garlic, two (2) cloves
- Lemon juice (fresh), five (5) tablespoons
- Parsley (a handful)
- Cayenne pepper (a pinch)
- Organic salt or sea salt (a pinch)
- Eggplant (700g)
- Sesame paste, six (6) tablespoons

Directions:

1. Firstly, it is necessary to preheat the oven to around 400 degrees Fahrenheit.
2. Wash the eggplants and use a fork to prick several places.
3. Place in the oven on a grid and heat for between thirty to forty minutes.
4. While this is going, chop the parsley and garlic and set aside.
5. Take off the eggplant from the oven after forty minutes and allow it to cool.
6. Once it's cooled, peel the eggplants and scoop out the pulp.
7. Chop the pulp finely on a chopping board and empty it in a mixing bowl.
8. In the mixing bowl, sprinkle the lemon juice and mash with a spoon until it becomes smooth.
9. Finally, add garlic, the parsley, and the sesame paste.
10. Season with pepper and salt to taste.
11. Serve.

Nutrition:

- Calories: 30
- Carbohydrates: 2 g
- Fat: 3 g
- Protein: 1g

84. Coriander Spread

Preparation Time: 14 minutes
Cooking Time: 16 minutes
Servings: 3
Ingredients:

- Chili (green), 1-2
- Ginger (fresh), ½ inch
- Lime juice (fresh), two (2) tablespoons
- Coconut flakes (freshly grated), one (1) cup
- Coriander leaves (fresh), three (3) cups
- Alkaline water, four (4) tablespoons
- Organic or sea salt, one pinch

Directions:

1. Chop the ginger, chili, and coriander leaves.
2. Include all elements in a blender machine and blend until the mix is smooth to consistency.

3. When that is done, you can add some organic or sea salt and season to taste.
4. Lastly, it is recommended that you put the mix in the fridge for about an hour.
5. Serve.

Nutrition:

- Calories: 22
- Carbohydrates: 2 g
- Fat: 43 g

85. Polo Salad Dressing

Preparation Time: 14 minutes
Cooking Time: 16 minutes
Servings: 3
Ingredients:

- Dates, two (2)
- Juice of lemon, (½ lemon)
- Alkaline water, ½ cup
- Cayenne pepper and sea salt, one (1) dash
- Extra virgin oil (cold-pressed), 1/3 cup
- Miso, one (1) tablespoon

Directions:

1. Include all elements in a blender machine and blast until the mix is smooth to consistency.
2. You can add additional salt and pepper if desired.
3. Serve.

Nutrition:

- Calories: 71
- Carbohydrates: 8g
- Fat: 3 g
- Protein: 2g

86. Citrus Alkaline Salad Dressing

Preparation Time: 14 minutes
Cooking Time: 16 minutes
Servings: 3
Ingredients:

- Garlic powder, one (1) teaspoon
- Rosemary (dried), ¼ teaspoon
- Cumin (ground), ½ teaspoon
- Oregano (ground), ½ teaspoon
- Basil (dried), one (1) teaspoon
- Olive oil (cold-pressed), ¾ cup
- Cayenne pepper and sea salt, one (1) dash
- Fresh lime or lemon juice, 1/3 cup

Directions:

1. Add all the ingredients in a mixer and blast until the mix is smooth to consistency.
2. You can season with pepper and salt if desired.
3. Serve.

Nutrition:

- Calories: 43
- Carbohydrates: 3 g
- Fat: 3 g

87. Avocado Spinach Dip

Preparation Time: 14 minutes
Cooking Time: 16 minutes
Servings: 3
Ingredients:

- Dill, one (1) cup
- Avocado, one (1)
- Garlic, one (1) clove
- Parsley, one (1) cup
- Spinach (fresh), 150g
- Tahini, one (1) tablespoon
- Chili, one (1)
- Pepper and sea salt to taste

Directions:

1. Include all elements in a blender machine
2. Blend until the mix turns creamy and smooth to consistency.
3. You can consist of pepper and salt to taste.
4. Serve.

Nutrition:

- Calories: 46
- Carbohydrates: 3g
- Fat: 3g
- Protein: 2g

88. Alkaline Vegetable Spread

Preparation Time: 14 minutes
Cooking Time: 16 minutes
Servings: 3
Ingredients:

- Pepper, one (1) pinch
- Tomato, one (1)
- Avocado, one (1)
- Yeast-free vegetable stock, one (1) teaspoon
- Bean sprouts, ½ cup
- Celery stalk, one (1)
- Alfalfa sprouts, ½ cup
- Sunflower seeds, one (1) handful
- Organic salt or sea salt, one (1) pinch
- Any garden herb of your choice, one (1) teaspoon
- Extra virgin oil (cold-pressed), one (1) tablespoon
- Cucumber ½

Directions:

1. Depending on how you like your spread, you can either blend it or not. Since we want this spread to be chunky, we won't Blend.
2. So, chop the alfalfa sprouts, cucumber, tomato, celery, and bean sprout into tiny pieces.
3. Get a mixing bowl and toss all the chopped ingredients into it.
4. Add sunflower seeds and mix properly.
5. Mash the avocado and add in a separate bowl, along with the olive oil, vegetable stock, lemon juice, salt and pepper, and herbs.
6. Stir until it forms a creamy paste.
7. Finally, mix the mashed avocado cream with the vegetables.
8. Stir consistently until all ingredients are mixed properly.
9. Refrigerate for about an hour.
10. Serve.

Nutrition:

- Calories: 12
- Carbohydrates: 1 g
- Fat: 7 g

89. Alkaline Sunflower Sauce

Preparation Time: 14 minutes
Cooking Time: 16 minutes
Servings: 3
Ingredients:

- Tomato, one (1)
- Sunflower seeds, 200g
- Red pepper, one (1)
- Garlic, one (1) clove
- Extra virgin olive oil (cold-pressed), one (teaspoon)
- Pepper (a pinch)
- Organic salt or sea salt (a pinch)
- Any herb of your choice

Directions:

1. Note: Before you start this process, you should soak the sunflower seeds for about four (4) hours before commencement.
2. Add all ingredients in a blender and

blast till the mix turns into a smooth cream.
3. Add your favourite herbs, pepper, and salt to taste.
4. Serve.

Nutrition:

- Calories: 200
- Protein: 7g

90. Almond-Red Bell Pepper Dip

Preparation Time: 14 minutes
Cooking Time: 16 minutes
Servings: 3
Ingredients:

- Garlic, 2-3 cloves
- Sea salt, one (1) pinch
- Cayenne pepper, one (1) pinch
- Extra virgin olive oil (cold-pressed), one (1) tablespoon
- Almonds, 60g
- Red bell pepper, 280g

Directions:

1. First of all, cook garlic and pepper until they are soft.
2. Add all ingredients in a mixer and blend until the mix becomes smooth and creamy.
3. Finally, add pepper and salt to taste.
4. Serve.

Nutrition:

- Calories: 51
- Carbohydrates: 10g
- Fat: 1g
- Protein: 2g

91. Hummus

Preparation Time: 14 minutes
Cooking Time: 16 minutes
Servings: 3
Ingredients:

- Olive oil (cold pressed), one (1) tablespoon
- Fresh Lemon juice, two (2) tablespoons
- Chili, one (1)
- Pepper and sea salt to taste
- Tahini, one (1) tablespoon
- Garlic (finely chopped), two (2) cloves
- Chickpeas (home-cooked), 300g-400g
- Vegetable broth (yeast-free), 50ml

Directions:

1. Blend all the ingredients until it becomes creamy and smooth.
2. Add pepper and salt to taste.
3. Serve.

Nutrition:

- Calories: 70
- Carbohydrates: 4g
- Fat: 5g
- Protein: 2 g

92. Sweet Barbecue Sauce

Preparation Time: 14 minutes
Cooking Time: 16 minutes
Servings: 3
Ingredients:

- 6 quartered plum tomatoes
- 1/4 cup of chopped white onions
- 1/4 cup of date sugar
- 2 teaspoons of pure sea salt
- 2 teaspoons agave syrup
- 1/4 teaspoon cayenne
- 2 teaspoons of onion powder
- 1/2 teaspoon ground ginger
- 1/8 teaspoon cloves

Directions:

1. Add all ingredients, excluding date sugar, to a blender and blend them

thoroughly. Pour mixture into a saucepan and add a date sugar. Cook over average heat, stirring occasionally to prevent sticking until boiling. Reduce heat to a simmer. Cover the saucepan with a lid and cook for 15 minutes, stirring from time to time.

2. Use an immersion blender to blend the sauce until it is smooth. Remain to cook at low heat until the sauce thickens for about 10 minutes. Allow mixture to cool before using it. Serve and enjoy your sweet barbecue sauce!

Nutrition:

- Calories: 30
- Carbohydrates: 4 g
- Fat: 1 g

93. Avocado Sauce

Preparation Time: 14 minutes
Cooking Time: 16 minutes
Servings: 3
Ingredients:

- 1 ripe avocado
- 1 pinch of basil
- ½ teaspoon of oregano
- 1/2 teaspoon of onion powder
- 2 teaspoons of minced onion
- 1/2 teaspoon of pure sea salt

Directions:

1. Cut the avocado in half, peel it and remove the seed. Slice it into small pieces and throw into a food processor. Add all other ingredients and blend for 2 to 3 minutes until smooth. Serve and enjoy your avocado sauce!

Nutrition:

- Calories: 14
- Carbohydrates: 2 g
- Protein: 1g

94. Fragrant Tomato Sauce

Preparation Time: 14 minutes
Cooking Time: 16 minutes
Servings: 3
Ingredients:

- 5 Roma tomatoes
- 1 pinch of basil
- 1 teaspoon of oregano
- 1 teaspoon of onion powder
- 2 teaspoon of minced onion
- 2 teaspoon agave syrup
- 1 teaspoon of pure sea salt
- 2 tablespoons of grape seed oil

Directions:

1. Make an X cut on the lowermost of the Roma tomatoes and place them into a pot of hot water for just 1 minute. Take away the tomatoes from the water using a spoon and shock them, placing them in cold water for 30 seconds. Take them out and immediately peel with your fingers or a knife. Put all the ingredients into a mixer or a food processor and blend for 1 minute until smooth. Serve and enjoy your fragrant tomato sauce.

Nutrition:

- Calories: 20
- Carbohydrates: 2 g
- Protein: 1g

95. Guacamole

Preparation Time: 14 minutes
Cooking Time: 16 minutes
Servings: 3
Ingredients:

- 1 minced Roma tomato
- 2 avocados

- 1/2 cup of chopped cilantro
- 1/2 cup of minced red onion
- 1/2 teaspoon of cayenne powder
- 1/2 teaspoon of onion powder
- 1/2 teaspoon of pure sea salt
- Juice from ½ lime

Directions:

1. Cut the avocados in half, peel, and remove the seeds. Slice into tiny pieces and put them in a medium bowl. Add all other ingredients, excluding the Roma tomato, to the bowl. Using a masher, mix together until becomes smooth. Add the minced Roma tomatoes to the mixture and mix well.
2. Serve and enjoy your delicious guacamole!

Nutrition:

- Calories: 12
- Fat: 1 g

96. Garlic Sauce

Preparation Time: 14 minutes
Cooking Time: 16 minutes
Servings: 3
Ingredients:

- 1/4 cup of diced shallots
- 1 tablespoon of onion powder
- 1/4 teaspoon of dill
- 1/2 teaspoon of ginger
- 1/2 teaspoon of pure sea salt
- 1 cup of grapeseed oil

Directions:

1. Find a glass jar with a lid. Put all ingredients for the sauce in the jar and shake them well. Place the sauce mixture in the refrigerator for at least 1 hour. Serve and enjoy your "garlic" sauce!

Nutrition:

- Calories: 48
- Carbohydrates: 2 g
- Fat: 4 g

97. Pesto Saucy Cream Recipe

Preparation Time: 14 minutes
Cooking Time: 16 minutes
Servings: 3
Ingredients:

- 1 small avocado (Hass)
- 1 cup walnuts
- 3 tablespoons sour orange or lime
- 1/8 teaspoon basil
- 1/4 teaspoon onion powder
- 1/4 teaspoon cayenne pepper
- 1 teaspoon spring water

Directions:

1. Make a slit with a knife lengthwise around the avocado. Split open the avocado into two. Then using your heavy knife carefully, hit down the avocado seed, turn and pull out the seed. Scoop out the avocado meat and remove the skin. Then, add all of the ingredients to your blender and blend until all of the ingredients are thoroughly mixed and becomes smooth.

Nutrition:

- Calories: 65
- Carbohydrates: 4 g
- Fat: 5 g
- Protein: 3 g

Chapter 7: Special Ingredients

98. Homemade Hemp Seed Milk

Preparation Time: 15 minutes
Cooking Time: 2 hours
Servings: 2 cups
Ingredients:

- 2 tablespoons of hemp seeds
- 2 tablespoons of agave syrup
- 1/8 teaspoon of pure sea salt
- 2 cups of spring water
- Fruits (optional)*

Directions:

1. Place all ingredients, except fruits, into the blender.
2. Blend them for two minutes.
3. Add fruits and repeatedly blend for 30 to 50 seconds.
4. Leave milk in a refrigerator until cold.
5. Enjoy your homemade hemp seed milk!

Nutrition:

- Calories: 83
- Carbohydrates: 1.3 g
- Protein: 4.7 g
- Fat: 7.3 g

99. Spicy Infused Oil

Preparation Time: 5 minutes
Cooking Time: 24 hours
Servings: 1 cup
Ingredients:

- 1 tablespoon of crushed cayenne pepper
- 3/4 cup of grapeseed oil

Directions:

1. Fill a glass jar with a lid or a squeeze bottle with grapeseed oil.
2. Add crushed cayenne pepper to the jar/bottle.
3. Shake it and let the oil infuse for at least 24 hours.
4. Add it to a dish and enjoy your spicy infused oil!

Nutrition:

- Calories: 120
- Fat: 14 g

100. Italian Infused Oil

Preparation Time: 5 minutes
Cooking Time: 24 hours
Servings: 1 cup
Ingredients:

- 1 teaspoon of oregano
- 1 teaspoon of basil
- 1 pinch of pure sea salt
- 3/4 cup of grapeseed oil

Directions:

1. Fill a glass jar with a lid or a squeeze bottle with grapeseed oil.
2. Mix seasoning together and add them to the jar/bottle.
3. Shake it and let the oil infuse for at least 24 hours.
4. Add it to a dish and enjoy your Italian infused oil!

Nutrition:

- Calories: 120
- Fat: 14 g

101. Garlic Infused Oil

Preparation Time: 5 minutes
Cooking Time: 24 hours
Servings: 1 cup
Ingredients:

- 1/2 teaspoon of dill
- 1/2 teaspoon of ginger powder
- 1 tablespoon of onion powder
- 1/2 teaspoon of pure sea salt

- 3/4 cup of grapeseed oil

Directions:

1. Fill a glass jar with a lid or a squeeze bottle with Grape Seed Oil.
2. Add the seasonings to the jar/bottle.
3. Shake it and let the oil infuse for at least 24 hours.
4. Add it to a dish and enjoy your "Garlic" Infused Oil!

Nutrition:

- Calories: 130
- Fat: 14 g

102. Papaya Seed Mango Dressing

Preparation Time: 5 minutes
Cooking Time: 10 minutes
Servings: 1/2 cups

Ingredients:

- 1 cup of chopped mango
- 1 teaspoon of ground papaya seeds
- 1 teaspoon of basil
- 1 teaspoon of onion powder
- 1 teaspoon of agave syrup
- 2 tablespoons of lime juice
- 1/4 cup of grapeseed oil
- 1/4 teaspoon of pure sea salt

Directions:

1. Prepare and place all ingredients into the blender.
2. Blend for one minute until smooth.
3. Add it to a salad and enjoy your papaya seed mango dressing!

Nutrition:

- Calories: 120
- Fat: 14 g

103. Tomato Ginger Dressing

Preparation Time: 5 minutes
Cooking Time: 10 minutes
Servings: 1/2 cups

Ingredients:

- 2 chopped plum tomatoes
- 1 teaspoon of minced ginger*
- 1 tablespoon of agave syrup
- 2 tablespoons of chopped onion
- 2 tablespoons of sesame seeds
- 1 tablespoon of lime juice

Directions:

1. Prepare and place all ingredients into the blender.
2. Blend for one minute until smooth.
3. Add it to a salad and enjoy your tomato ginger dressing!

Nutrition:

- Calories: 40.3
- Fat: 4.1 g
- Fiber: 0.1 g

104. Dill Cucumber Dressing

Preparation Time: 5 minutes
Cooking Time: 10 minutes
Servings: 1/2 cups

Ingredients:

- 1 teaspoon of fresh dill*
- 1 cup of quartered cucumbers
- 1/2 teaspoon of onion powder
- 2 teaspoons of agave syrup
- 1 tablespoon of lime juice
- 1/4 cup of Avocado oil

Directions:

1. Prepare and place all ingredients into the blender.
2. Blend for one minute until smooth.
3. Add it to a salad and enjoy your dill cucumber dressing!

Nutrition:

- Calories: 60
- Carbohydrates: 3 g
- Fat: 5

105. Homemade Walnut Milk

Preparation Time: 15 minutes
Cooking Time: Minimum 8 hours
Servings: 4 cups
Ingredients:

- 1 cup of raw walnuts
- 1/8 teaspoon of pure sea salt
- 3 cups of spring water + extra for soaking

Directions:

1. Put raw walnuts in a small pot and cover them with three inches of water.
2. Soak the walnuts for at least eight hours.
3. Drain and rinse the walnuts with cold water.
4. Add the soaked walnuts, pure sea salt, and three cups of spring water to a blender.
5. Mix well until smooth.
6. Strain it if you need to.
7. Enjoy your homemade walnut milk!

Nutrition:

- Calories: 200
- Carbohydrate: 3.89 gr
- Sugar: 1 g
- Fiber: 2 g
- Protein: 5 g
- Fat: 20

106. Aquafaba

Preparation Time: 15 minutes
Cooking Time: 2 Hours 30 Minutes
Servings: 2-4 Cups
Ingredients:

- 1 bag of garbanzo beans
- 1 teaspoon of pure sea salt
- 6 cups of spring water + extra for soaking

Directions:

1. Place garbanzo beans in a large pot, add spring water and pure sea salt. Bring to a rolling boil.
2. Remove from the heat and leave to soak kindly for 30 to 40 minutes.
3. Strain garbanzo beans and add 6 cups of spring water.
4. Boil for 1 hour and 30 minutes on medium heat.
5. Strain the garbanzo beans. This strained water is Aquafaba.
6. Pour Aquafaba into a glass jar with a lid and place it into the refrigerator.
7. After cooling, Aquafaba becomes thicker. If it is too liquid, repeatedly boil for 10-20 minutes.

Useful tips:

- Aquafaba is a good alternative for an egg:
- 2 tablespoons of Aquafaba = 1 egg white
- 3 tablespoons of Aquafaba = 1 egg.

Nutrition:

- Calories: 46
- Carbs: 8 g
- Fiber: 2 g
- Protein: 3 g

Chapter 8: Snacks & Bread

107. Spinach and Sesame Crackers

Preparation Time: 5 minutes
Cooking Time: 15 minutes
Servings: 4
Ingredients:

- 2 tablespoons white sesame seeds
- 1 cup fresh spinach, washed
- 1 2/3 cups of all-purpose flour
- 1/2 cup of water
- 1/2 teaspoon baking powder
- 1 teaspoon olive oil
- 1 teaspoon of salt

Directions:

1. Transfer the spinach to a blender with a half cup of water and blend until smooth.
2. Add 2 tablespoons white sesame seeds, ½ teaspoon baking powder, 1 2/3 cups all-purpose flour, and 1 teaspoon salt to a bowl and stir well until combined. Add in 1 teaspoon olive oil and spinach water. Mix again and knead by using your hands until you obtain a smooth dough.
3. If the made dough is too gluey, then add more flour.
4. Using your parchment paper lightly roll out the dough as thin as possible. Cut into squares with a pizza cutter.
5. Bake into a preheated oven at 400° for about 15to 20 minutes. Once done, let cool and then serve.

Nutrition:

- 223 calories
- 3g fat
- 41g total carbohydrates
- 6g protein

108. Mini Nacho Pizzas

Preparation Time: 5 minutes
Cooking Time: 10 minutes
Servings: 4
Ingredients:

- 1/4 cup refried beans, vegan
- 2 tablespoons tomato, diced
- 2 English muffins, split in half
- 1/4 cup onion, sliced
- 1/3 cup vegan cheese, shredded
- 1 small jalapeno, sliced
- 1/3 cup roasted tomato salsa
- 1/2 avocado, diced and tossed in lemon juice

Directions:

1. Add the refried beans/salsa onto the muffin bread. Sprinkle with shredded vegan cheese followed by the veggie toppings.
2. Transfer to a baking sheet and place in a preheated oven at 350 to 400 F on a top rack.
3. Put into the oven for 10 minutes and then broil for 2minutes, so that the top becomes bubbly.
4. Take out from the oven and let them cool at room temperature.
5. Top with avocado. Enjoy!

Nutrition:

- 133 calories
- 4.2g fat
- 719g total carbohydrates
- 6g protein

109. Pizza Sticks

Preparation Time: 10 minutes
Cooking Time: 30 minutes
Servings: 16 sticks
Ingredients:

- 5 tablespoons tomato sauce
- Few pinches of dried basil
- 1 block extra firm tofu
- 2 tablespoon + 2 teaspoon nutritional yeast

Directions:

1. Cape the tofu in a paper tissue and put a cutting board on top, place something heavy on top and drain for about 10 to 15 minutes.
2. In the meantime, line your baking sheet with parchment paper. Cut the tofu into 16 equal pieces and place them on a baking sheet.
3. Spread each pizza stick with a teaspoon of marinara sauce.
4. Sprinkle each stick with a half teaspoon of yeast, followed by basil on top.
5. Bake into a preheated oven at 425 F for about 28 to 30 minutes. Serve and enjoy!

Nutrition:

- 33 calories
- 1.7g fat
- 2g total carbs
- 3g protein

110. Raw Broccoli Poppers

Preparation Time: 2 minutes
Cooking Time: 8 minutes
Servings: 4
Ingredients:

- 1/8 cup of water
- 1/8 teaspoon of fine sea salt
- 4 cups broccoli florets, washed and cut into 1-inch pieces
- 1/4 teaspoon turmeric powder
- 1 cup unsalted cashews, soaked overnight or at least 3-4 hours and drained
- 1/4 teaspoon onion powder
- 1 red bell pepper, seeded and
- 2 heaping tablespoons nutritional
- 2 tablespoons lemon juice

Directions:

1. Transfer the drained cashews to a high-speed blender and pulse for about 30 seconds. Add in the chopped pepper and pulse again for 30 seconds.
2. Add some 2 tablespoons of lemon juice, 1/8 cup of water, 2 heaping tablespoons of nutritional yeast, ¼ teaspoon of onion powder, 1/8 teaspoon of fine sea salt, and 1/4 teaspoon of turmeric powder. Pulse for about 45 seconds until smooth.
3. Handover the broccoli into a bowl and add in chopped cheesy cashew mixture. Toss well until coated.
4. Transfer the pieces of broccoli to the trays of a yeast dehydrator.
5. Follow the dehydrator's instructions and dehydrate for about 8 minutes at 125 F or until crunchy.

Nutrition:

- 408 calories, 32g fat
- 22g total carbohydrates
- 15g protein

111. Blueberry Cauliflower

Preparation Time: 2 minutes
Cooking Time: 5 minutes
Servings: 1
Ingredients:

- ¼ cup of frozen strawberries

- 2 teaspoons maple syrup
- ¾ cup unsweetened cashew milk
- 1 teaspoon vanilla extract
- ½ cup of plain cashew yogurt
- 5 tablespoons powdered peanut butter
- ¾ cup of frozen wild blueberries
- ½ cup of cauliflower florets, coarsely chopped

Directions:

1. Add all the smoothie ingredients to a high-speed blender.
2. Blitz to combine until smooth.
3. Pour into a chilled glass and serve.

Nutrition:

- 340 calories
- 11g fat
- 48g total carbohydrates
- 16g protein

112. Candied Ginger

Preparation Time: 10 minutes
Cooking Time: 40 minutes
Servings: 3 to 5
Ingredients:

- 2 1/2 cups salted pistachios, shelled
- 1 1/4 teaspoons powdered ginger
- 3 tablespoons pure maple syrup

Directions:

1. Add 1 1/4 teaspoons powdered ginger to a bowl with pistachios. Stir well until combined. There should be no lumps.
2. Drizzle with 3 tablespoons of maple syrup and stir well.
3. Transfer to a baking sheet lined with parchment paper and spread evenly.
4. Cook into a preheated oven at 275 F for about 20 minutes.
5. Take out from the oven, stir, and cook for further 10 to 15 minutes.
6. Let it cool for about a few minutes until crispy. Enjoy!

Nutrition:

- 378 calories
- 27.6g fat
- 26g total carbohydrates
- 13g protein

113. Chia Crackers

Preparation Time: 20 minutes
Cooking Time: 1 hour
Servings: 24-26 crackers
Ingredients:

- 1/2 cup of pecans, chopped
- 1/2 cup of chia seeds
- 1/2 teaspoon cayenne pepper
- 1 cup of water
- 1/4 cup of nutritional yeast
- 1/2 cup of pumpkin seeds
- 1/4 cup of ground flax
- Salt and pepper, to taste

Directions:

1. Mix around 1/2 cup chia seeds and 1 cup water. Keep it aside.
2. Take another bowl and combine all the remaining ingredients. Combine well and stir in the chia water mixture until you obtained dough.
3. Transfer the dough onto a baking sheet and rollout (¼" thick).
4. Transfer into a preheated oven at 325°F and bake for about half an hour.
5. Take out from the oven, flip over the dough, and cut it into desired cracker shape/squares.
6. Spread and back again for a further half an hour, or until crispy and browned.
7. Once done, take out from the oven and let them cool at room

temperature. Enjoy!

Nutrition:

- 41 calories
- 3.1g fat
- 2g total carbohydrates
- 2g protein

114. Orange- Spiced Pumpkin Hummus

Preparation Time: 2 minutes
Cooking Time: 5 minutes
Servings: 4 cups
Ingredients:

- 1 tablespoon maple syrup
- 1/2 teaspoon salt
- 1 can (16oz.) garbanzo beans,
- 1/8 teaspoon ginger or nutmeg
- 1 cup of canned pumpkin
- 1/8 teaspoon cinnamon
- 1/4 cup of tahini
- 1 tablespoon fresh orange juice
- A pinch of orange zest, for garnish
- 1 tablespoon apple cider vinegar

Directions:

1. Mix all the ingredients to a food processor blender and blend until slightly chunky.
2. Serve right away and enjoy it!

Nutrition:

- 291 calories
- 22.9g fat
- 15g total carbohydrates
- 12g protein

115. Cinnamon Maple Sweet Potato Bites

Preparation Time: 5 minutes
Cooking Time: 25 minutes
Servings: 3 to 4

Ingredients:

- ½ teaspoon corn-starch
- 1 teaspoon cinnamon
- 4 medium sweet potatoes, then peeled, and cut into bite-size cubes
- 2 to 3 tablespoons maple syrup
- 3 tablespoons butter, melted

Directions:

1. Transfer the potato cubes to a Ziploc bag and add in 3 tablespoons of melted butter. Seal and shake well until the potato cubes are coated with butter.
2. Add in the remaining ingredients and shake again.
3. Transfer the potato cubes to a parchment-lined baking sheet. Cubes shouldn't be stacked on one another.
4. Sprinkle with cinnamon, if needed, and bake in a preheated oven at 425°F for about 25 to 30 minutes, stirring once during cooking.
5. Once done, take them out and stand at room temperature. Enjoy!

Nutrition:

- 436 calories
- 17.4g fat
- 71.8g total carbohydrates
- 4.1g protein

116. Cheesy Kale Chips

Preparation Time: 3 minutes
Cooking Time: 12 minutes
Servings: 4
Ingredients:

- 3 tablespoons nutritional yeast
- 1 head curly kale, washed, ribs
- 3/4 teaspoon garlic powder
- 1 tablespoon olive oil
- 1 teaspoon onion powder
- Salt, to taste

Directions:

1. Line cookie sheets with parchment paper.
2. Drain the kale leaves and spread on a paper removed and leaves torn into a chip-towel. Then, kindly transfer the leaves to a bowl and sized pieces. Add in 1 teaspoon of onion powder, 3 tablespoons of nutritional yeast, 1 tablespoon of olive oil, and ¾ teaspoon of garlic powder. Mix with your hands.
3. Spread the kale onto prepared cookie sheets. They shouldn't touch each other.
4. Bake into a preheated oven for about 350 F for about 10 to 12 minutes.
5. Once crisp, take out from the oven, and sprinkle with a bit of salt. Serve and enjoy!

Nutrition:

- 71 calories
- 4g fat
- 5g total carbohydrates
- 4g protein

117. Lemon Roasted Bell Pepper

Preparation Time: 10 minutes
Cooking Time: 5 minutes
Servings: 4
Ingredients:

- 4 bell peppers
- 1 teaspoon olive oil
- 1 tablespoon mango juice
- 1/4 teaspoon garlic, minced
- 1 teaspoons oregano
- 1 pinch of salt
- 1 pinch of pepper

Directions:

1. Start heating the Air Fryer to 390 degrees F.
2. Place some bell pepper in the air fryer.
3. Drizzle it with the olive oil and air fry for 5 minutes.
4. Take a serving plate and transfer it.
5. Take a small bowl and add garlic, oregano, mango juice, salt, and pepper.
6. Mix them well and drizzle the mixture over the peppers.
7. Serve and enjoy!

Nutrition:

- Calories: 59 kcal
- Carbohydrates: 6 g
- Fat: 5 g
- Protein: 4 g

118. Subtle Roasted Mushrooms

Preparation Time: 10 minutes
Cooking Time: 5 minutes
Servings: 4
Ingredients:

- 2 teaspoons mixed Sebi Friendly herbs
- 1 tablespoon olive oil

- 1/2 teaspoon garlic powder
- 2 pounds' mushrooms
- 2 tablespoons date sugar

Directions:

1. Wash mushrooms and turn dry in a plate of mixed greens spinner.
2. Quarter and put them in a safe spot.
3. Put garlic, oil, and spices in the dish of your oar type air fryer.
4. Warmth for 2 minutes.
5. Stir it.
6. Add some mushrooms and cook 25 minutes.
7. Then include vermouth and cook for 5 minutes more.
8. Serve and enjoy!

Nutrition:

- Calories: 94 kcal
- Carbohydrates: 3 g
- Fat: 8 g
- Protein: 2 g

119. Fancy Spelt Bread

Preparation Time: 10 minutes
Cooking Time: 5 minutes
Servings: 4
Ingredients:

- 1 cup spring water
- 1/2 cup of coconut milk
- 3 tablespoons avocado oil
- 1 teaspoon baking soda
- 1 tablespoon agave nectar
- 4 and 1/2 cups spelt flour
- 1 and 1/2 teaspoon salt

Directions:

1. Preheat your Air Fryer to 355 degrees F.
2. Take a big bowl and add baking soda, salt, flour whisk well.
3. Add 3/4 cup of water, plus coconut milk, oil, and mix well.
4. Sprinkle your working surface with flour, add dough to the flour.
5. Roll well.
6. Knead for about three minutes, adding small amounts of flour until dough is a nice ball.
7. Place parchment paper in your cooking basket.
8. Lightly grease your pan and put the dough inside.
9. Transfer into Air Fryer and bake for 30-45 minutes until done.
10. Remove then insert a stick to check for doneness.
11. If done already serve and enjoy, if not, let it cook for a few minutes more.

Nutrition:

- Calories: 203 kcal
- Carbohydrates: 37 g
- Fat: 4g
- Protein: 7 g

120. Crispy Crunchy Hummus

Preparation Time: 10 minutes
Cooking Time: 10-15 minutes
Servings: 4
Ingredients:

- 1/2 a red onion
- 2 tablespoons fresh coriander
- 1/4 cup of cherry tomatoes
- 1/2 a red bell pepper
- 1 tablespoon dulse flakes
- Juice of lime
- Salt to taste
- 3 tablespoons olive oil
- 2 tablespoons tahini
- 1 cup of warm chickpeas

Directions:

- Prepare your Air Fryer cooking basket
- Add chickpeas to your cooking

container and cook for 10-15 minutes, making a point to continue blending them every once in a while until they are altogether warmed

- Add warmed chickpeas to a bowl and include tahini, salt, lime
- Utilize a fork to pound chickpeas and fixings in glue until smooth
- Include hacked onion, cherry tomatoes, ringer pepper, dulse drops, and olive oil
- Blend well until consolidated
- Serve hummus with a couple of cuts of spelt bread

Nutrition:

- Calories: 95 kcal
- Carbohydrates: 5 g
- Fat: 5 g
- Protein: 5 g

121. Chick Pea and Kale Dish

Preparation Time: 10 minutes
Cooking Time: 25-30 minutes
Servings: 4
Ingredients:

- 2 cups chickpea flour
- 1/2 cup green bell pepper, diced
- 1/2 cup onions, minced
- 1 tablespoon oregano
- 1 tablespoon salt
- 1 teaspoon cayenne
- 4 cups spring water
- 2 tablespoons grapeseed oil

Directions:

1. Boil spring water in a large pot.
2. Lower heat into medium and whisk in chickpea flour.
3. Add some minced onions, diced green bell pepper, seasoning to the pot and cook for 10 minutes.
4. Cover dish using a baking sheet, grease with oil.
5. Pour batter into the sheet and spread with a spatula.
6. Cover with another sheet.
7. Transfer to a fridge and chill, for 20 minutes.
8. Remove from the freezer and cut the batter into fry shapes.
9. Preheat the Air Fryer to 385 degrees F.
10. Transfer fries into the cooking basket, lightly greased, and cover with parchment.
11. Bake for about 15 minutes, flip and bake for 10 minutes more until golden brown.
12. Serve and enjoy!

Nutrition:

- Calories: 271 kcal
- Carbohydrates: 28 g
- Fat: 15 g
- Protein: 9 g

122. Zucchini Chips

Preparation Time: 10 minutes
Cooking Time: 12-15 minutes
Servings: 4
Ingredients:

- Salt to taste
- Grapeseed oil as needed
- 6 zucchinis

Directions:

1. Preheat the Air Fryer to 330 F.
2. Wash zucchini, slice zucchini into thin strips.
3. Put slices in a bowl and add oil, salt, and toss.
4. Spread over the cooking basket, fry for 12-15 minutes.

5. Serve and enjoy!

Nutrition:

- Calories: 92 kcal
- Carbohydrates: 6 g
- Fat: 7 g
- Protein: 2 g

123. Classic Blueberry Spelt Muffins

Preparation Time: 10 minutes
Cooking Time: 12-15 minutes
Servings: 4
Ingredients:

- 1/4 sea salt
- 1/3 cup of maple syrup
- 1 teaspoon baking powder
- 1/2 cup of sea moss
- 3/4 cup of spelt flour
- 3/4 cup of Kamut flour
- 1 cup of hemp milk
- 1 cup of blueberries

Directions:

1. Preheat Air Fryer to 380 degrees F.
2. Take your muffin tins and gently grease them.
3. Take a bowl and add flour, syrup, salt, baking powder, seamless, and mix well.
4. Add milk and mix well.
5. Fold in blueberries.
6. Pour into muffin tins.
7. Transfer to the cooking basket, bake for 20-25 minutes until nicely baked.
8. Serve and enjoy!

Nutrition:

- Calories: 217 kcal,
- Carbohydrates: 32 g
- Fat: 9 g
- Protein: 4 g

124. Genuine Healthy Crackers

Preparation Time: 10 minutes
Cooking Time: 12-15 minutes
Servings: 4
Ingredients:

- 1/2 cup of Rye flour
- 1 cup of spelt flour
- 2 teaspoons sesame seed
- 1 teaspoon agave syrup
- 1 teaspoon salt
- 2 tablespoons grapeseed oil
- 3/4 cup of spring water

Directions:

1. Preheat the Air Fryer to 330 degrees F.
2. Take a medium bowl and add all ingredients, mix well.
3. Make dough ball.
4. Prepare a place for rolling out the dough, cover with a piece of parchment.
5. Lightly grease the paper with grape seed oil, place dough.
6. Roll out, dough with a rolling pin, add more flour if needed.
7. Take a shape cutter and cut dough into squares.
8. Place squares in the Air Fryer cooking basket.
9. Brush with more oil.
10. Sprinkle salt.
11. Bake for 10-15 minutes until golden.
12. Let it cool, serve, and enjoy!

Nutrition:

- Calories: 226 kcal
- Carbohydrates: 41 g
- Fat: 3 g
- Protein: 11 g

125. Dr. Sebi's Tortilla Chips

Preparation Time: 10 minutes
Cooking Time: 8-12 minutes
Servings: 4
Ingredients:

- 2 cups of spelt flour
- 1 teaspoon of salt
- 1/2 cup of spring water
- 1/3 cup of grapeseed oil

Directions:

1. Preheat your Air Fryer into 320 degrees F.
2. Take the food processor then add salt, flour, and process well for 15 seconds.
3. Gradually add grapeseed oil until mixed.
4. Keep mixing until you have a nice dough.
5. Formulate work surface and cover in a piece of parchment, sprinkle flour.
6. Knead the dough for 1-2 minutes.
7. Grease cooking basket with oil.
8. Transfer dough on the cooking basket, brush oil and sprinkle salt.
9. Cut dough into 8 triangles.
10. Bake for about 8-12 minutes until golden brown.
11. Serve and enjoy once done!

Nutrition:

- Calories: 288 kcal
- Carbohydrates: 18 g
- Fat: 17 g
- Protein: 16 g

126. Pumpkin Spice Crackers

Preparation Time: 10 minutes
Cooking Time: 60 minutes
Servings: 06
Ingredients:

- 1⁄3 cup of coconut flour
- 2 tablespoons pumpkin pie spice
- 3⁄4 cup of sunflower seeds
- 3⁄4 cup of flaxseed
- 1⁄3 cup of sesame seeds
- 1 tablespoon ground psyllium husk powder
- 1 teaspoon of sea salt
- 3 tablespoons coconut oil, melted
- 11⁄3 cups of alkaline water

Directions:

1. Set your oven to 300 degrees F.
2. Combine all dry ingredients in a bowl.
3. Add water and oil to the mixture and mix well.
4. Let the dough stay for 2 to 3 minutes.
5. Spread the dough evenly on a cookie sheet lined with parchment paper.
6. Bake for 30 minutes.
7. Reduce the oven heat to low and bake for another 30 minutes.
8. Crack the bread into bite-size pieces.
9. Serve

Nutrition:

- Calories 248
- Total Fat 15.7 g
- Saturated Fat 2.7 g
- Cholesterol 75 mg
- Sodium 94 mg
- Total Carbs 0.4 g
- Fiber 0g
- Sugar 0 g
- Protein 24.9 g

127. Spicy Roasted Nuts

Preparation Time: 10 minutes
Cooking Time: 15 minutes
Servings: 4
Ingredients:

- 8 oz. pecans or almonds or walnuts
- 1 teaspoon of sea salt
- 1 tablespoon of olive oil or coconut oil

- 1 teaspoon of ground cumin
- 1 teaspoon of paprika powder or chili powder

Directions:

1. Add all the ingredients to a skillet.
2. Roast the nuts until golden brown.
3. Serve and enjoy.

Nutrition:

- Calories 287
- Total Fat 29.5 g
- Saturated Fat 3 g
- Cholesterol 0 mg
- Total Carbs 5.9 g
- Sugar 1.4g
- Fiber 4.3 g
- Sodium 388 mg
- Protein 4.2 g

128. Wheat Crackers

Preparation Time: 10 minutes
Cooking Time: 20 minutes
Servings: 4
Ingredients:

- 1 3/4 cups almond flour
- 1 1/2 cups coconut flour
- 3/4 teaspoon of sea salt
- 1/3 cup of vegetable oil
- 1 cup of alkaline water
- Sea salt for sprinkling

Directions:

1. Set your oven to 350 degrees F.
2. Mix coconut flour, almond flour, and salt in a bowl.
3. Stir in vegetable oil and water. Mix well until smooth.
4. Spread this dough on a floured surface into a thin sheet.
5. Cut small squares out of this sheet.
6. Arrange the dough squares on a baking sheet lined with parchment paper.
7. For about 20 minutes, bake until it turns light golden.
8. Serve.

Nutrition:

- Calories 64
- Total Fat 9.2 g
- Saturated Fat 2.4 g
- Cholesterol 110 mg
- Sodium 276 mg
- Total Carbs 9.2 g
- Fiber 0.9 g
- Sugar 1.4 g
- Protein 1.5 g

129. Potato Chips

Preparation Time: 10 minutes
Cooking Time: 20 minutes
Servings: 4
Ingredients:

- 1 tablespoon vegetable oil
- 1 potato, sliced paper-thin
- Sea salt, to taste

Directions:

1. Toss potato with oil and sea salt.
2. Spread the slices in a baking dish in a single layer.
3. Cook in a microwave for 5 minutes until golden brown.
4. Serve.

Nutrition:

- Calories 80
- Total Fat 3.5 g
- Saturated Fat 0.1 g
- Cholesterol 320 mg
- Sodium 350 mg
- Total Carbs 11.6 g
- Fiber 0.7 g
- Sugar 0.7 g
- Protein 1.2 g

130. Zucchini Pepper Chips

Preparation Time: 10 minutes
Cooking Time: 15 minutes
Servings: 04
Ingredients:

- 1 2/3 cups vegetable oil
- 1 teaspoon garlic powder
- 1 teaspoon onion powder
- 1/2 teaspoon black pepper
- 3 tablespoons crushed red pepper flakes
- 2 zucchinis, thinly sliced

Directions:

1. Mix oil with all the spices in a bowl.
2. Add zucchini slices and mix well.
3. Transfer the mixture to a Ziplock bag and seal it.
4. Refrigerate for 10 minutes.
5. Spread the zucchini slices on a greased baking sheet.
6. Bake for 15 minutes
7. Serve.

Nutrition:

- Calories 172
- Total Fat 11.1 g
- Saturated Fat 5.8 g
- Cholesterol 610 mg
- Sodium 749 mg
- Total Carbs 19.9 g
- Fiber 0.2 g
- Sugar 0.2 g
- Protein 13.5 g

131. Apple Chips

Preparation Time: 5 minutes
Cooking Time: 45 minutes
Servings: 4
Ingredients:

- 2 Golden Delicious apples, cored and thinly sliced
- 1 1/2 teaspoons white sugar
- 1/2 teaspoon ground cinnamon

Directions:

1. Set your oven to 225 degrees F.
2. Place apple slices on a baking sheet.
3. Sprinkle sugar and cinnamon over apple slices.
4. Bake for 45 minutes.
5. Serve

Nutrition:

- Calories 127
- Total Fat 3.5 g
- Saturated Fat 0.5 g
- Cholesterol 162 mg
- Sodium 142 mg
- Total Carbs 33.6g
- Fiber 0.4 g
- Sugar 0.5 g
- Protein 4.5 g

132. Kale Crisps

Preparation Time: 10 minutes
Cooking Time: 10 minutes
Servings: 04
Ingredients:

- 1 bunch kale, remove the stems, leaves torn into even pieces
- 1 tablespoon of olive oil
- 1 teaspoon of sea salt

Directions:

1. Set your oven to 350 degrees F. Layer a baking sheet with parchment paper.
2. Spread the kale leaves on a paper towel to absorb all the moisture.
3. Toss the leaves with sea salt and olive oil.
4. Kindly spread them on the baking sheet and bake for 10 minutes.
5. Serve.

Nutrition:

- Calories 113

- Total Fat 7.5 g
- Saturated Fat 1.1 g
- Cholesterol 20 mg
- Sodium 97 mg
- Total Carbs 1.4 g
- Fiber 0 g
- Sugar 0 g
- Protein 1.1g

133. Carrot Chips

Preparation Time: 5 minutes
Cooking Time: 12 minutes
Servings: 4
Ingredients:

- 4 carrots, washed, peeled and sliced
- 2 teaspoons of extra-virgin olive oil
- 1/4 teaspoon of sea salt

Directions:

1. Set your oven to 350 degrees F.
2. Toss carrots with salt and olive oil.
3. Spread the slices into two baking sheets in a single layer.
4. Bake for 6 minutes on the upper and lower rack of the oven.
5. Switch the baking racks and bake for another 6 minutes.
6. Serve.

Nutrition:

- Calories 153
- Total Fat 7.5 g
- Saturated Fat 1.1 g
- Cholesterol 20 mg
- Sodium 97 mg
- Total Carbs 20.4 g
- Fiber 0 g
- Sugar 0 g
- Protein 3.1g

134. Pita Chips

Preparation Time: 5 minutes
Cooking Time: 12 minutes
Servings: 4
Ingredients:

- 12 pita bread pockets, sliced into triangles
- 1/2 cup olive oil
- 1/2 teaspoon ground black pepper
- 1 teaspoon of garlic salt
- 1/2 teaspoon dried basil
- 1 teaspoon dried chervil

Directions:

1. Set your oven to 400 degrees F.
2. Toss pita with all the remaining ingredients in a bowl.
3. Spread the seasoned triangles on a baking sheet.
4. Bake for 7 minutes until golden brown.
5. Serve with your favourite hummus.

Nutrition:

- Calories 201
- Total Fat 5.5 g
- Saturated Fat 2.1 g
- Cholesterol 10 mg
- Sodium 597 mg
- Total Carbs 2.4 g
- Fiber 0 g
- Sugar 0 g
- Protein 3.1g

135. Sweet Potato Chips

Preparation Time: 5 minutes
Cooking Time: 5 minutes
Servings: 4
Ingredients:

- 1 sweet potato, thinly sliced
- 2 teaspoons olive oil, or as needed
- Coarse sea salt, to taste

Directions:

1. Toss sweet potato with oil and salt.
2. Spread the slices in a baking dish in a single layer.
3. Cook in a microwave for 5 minutes until golden brown.
4. Serve.

Nutrition:

- Calories 213
- Total Fat 8.5 g
- Saturated Fat 3.1 g
- Cholesterol 120 mg
- Sodium 497 mg
- Total Carbs 21.4 g
- Fiber 0 g
- Sugar 0 g
- Protein 0.1g

Chapter 9: Desserts

136. Chocolate Crunch Bars

Preparation Time: 5 minutes
Cooking Time: 5 minutes
Servings: 4
Ingredients:

- 1 1/2 cups sugar-free chocolate chips
- 1 cup almond butter
- Stevia to taste
- 1/4 cup coconut oil
- 3 cups pecans, chopped

Directions:

1. Layer an 8-inch baking pan with parchment paper.
2. Mix chocolate chips with butter, coconut oil, and sweetener in a bowl.
3. Melt it by heating in a microwave for 2 to 3 minutes until well mixed.
4. Stir in nuts and seeds. Mix gently.
5. Pour this batter carefully into the baking pan and spread evenly.
6. Refrigerate for 2 to 3 hours.
7. Slice and serve.

Nutrition:

- Calories 316
- Total Fat 30.9 g
- Saturated Fat 8.1 g
- Cholesterol 0 mg
- Total Carbs 8.3 g
- Sugar 1.8 g
- Fiber 3.8 g
- Sodium 8 mg
- Protein 6.4 g

137. Homemade Protein Bar

Preparation Time: 5 minutes
Cooking Time: 10 minutes
Servings: 4
Ingredients:

- 1 cup nut butter
- 4 tablespoons coconut oil
- 2 scoops vanilla protein
- Stevia, to taste
- ½ teaspoon of sea salt

Optional Ingredients:

- 1 teaspoon cinnamon

Directions:

1. Mix coconut oil with butter, protein, stevia, and salt in a dish.
2. Stir in cinnamon and chocolate chip.
3. Press the mixture firmly and freeze until firm.
4. Cut the crust into small bars.
5. Serve and enjoy.

Nutrition:

- Calories 179
- Total Fat 15.7 g
- Saturated Fat 8 g
- Cholesterol 0 mg
- Total Carbs 4.8 g
- Sugar 3.6 g
- Fiber 0.8 g
- Sodium 43 mg
- Protein 5.6 g

138. Shortbread Cookies

Preparation Time: 10 minutes
Cooking Time: 70 minutes
Servings: 6
Ingredients:

- 2 1/2 cups almond flour
- 6 tablespoons nut butter
- 1/2 cup erythritol
- 1 teaspoon vanilla essence

Directions:

1. Preheat your oven to 350 degrees F.
2. Layer a cookie sheet with parchment paper.
3. Beat butter with erythritol until fluffy.
4. Stir in vanilla essence and almond flour. Mix well until becomes crumbly.
5. Spoon out a tablespoon of cookie dough onto the cookie sheet.
6. Add more dough to make as many cookies.
7. Bake for 15 minutes until brown.
8. Serve.

Nutrition:

- Calories 288
- Total Fat 25.3 g
- Saturated Fat 6.7 g
- Cholesterol 23 mg
- Total Carbs 9.6 g
- Sugar 0.1 g
- Fiber 3.8 g
- Sodium 74 mg
- Potassium 3 mg
- Protein 7.6 g

139. Coconut Chip Cookies

Preparation Time: 10 minutes
Cooking Time: 15 minutes
Servings: 4
Ingredients:

- 1 cup almond flour
- ½ cup cacao nibs
- ½ cup coconut flakes, unsweetened
- 1/3 cup erythritol
- ½ cup almond butter
- ¼ cup nut butter, melted
- ¼ cup almond milk
- Stevia, to taste
- ¼ teaspoon of sea salt

Directions:

1. Preheat your oven to 350 degrees F.
2. Layer a cookie sheet with parchment paper.
3. Add and then combine all the dry ingredients in a glass bowl.
4. Whisk in butter, almond milk, vanilla essence, stevia, and almond butter.
5. Beat well, then stir in the dry mixture. Mix well.
6. Spoon out a tablespoon of cookie dough on the cookie sheet.
7. Add more dough to make as many as 16 cookies.
8. Flatten each cookie using your fingers.
9. Bake for 25 minutes until golden brown.
10. Let them sit for 15 minutes.
11. Serve.

Nutrition:

- Calories 192
- Total Fat 17.44 g
- Saturated Fat 11.5 g
- Cholesterol 125 mg
- Total Carbs 2.2 g
- Sugar 1.4 g

- Fiber 2.1 g
- Sodium 135 mg
- Protein 4.7 g

140. Peanut Butter Bars

Preparation Time: 10 minutes
Cooking time: 10 minutes
Servings: 6
Ingredients:

- 3/4 cup almond flour
- 2 oz. almond butter
- 1/4 cup Swerve
- 1/2 cup peanut butter
- 1/2 teaspoon vanilla

Directions:

1. Combine all the ingredients for bars.
2. Transfer this mixture to a 6-inch small pan. Press it firmly.
3. Refrigerate for 30 minutes.
4. Slice and serve.

Nutrition:

- Calories 214
- Total Fat 19 g
- Saturated Fat 5.8 g
- Cholesterol 15 mg
- Total Carbs 6.5 g
- Sugar 1.9 g
- Fiber 2.1 g
- Sodium 123 mg
- Protein 6.5 g

141. Zucchini Bread Pancakes

Preparation Time: 15 minutes
Cooking Time: 35 minutes
Servings: 3
Ingredients:

- Grape seed oil, 1 tbsp.
- Chopped walnuts, .5 c
- Walnut milk, 2 c
- Shredded zucchini, 1 c
- Mashed burro banana, .25 c
- Date sugar, 2 tbsp.
- Kamut flour or spelt, 2 c

Directions:

1. Place the date sugar and flour into a bowl. Whisk together.
2. Add in the mashed banana and walnut milk. Stir until combined. Remember to scrape the bowl to get all the dry mixture. Add in walnuts and zucchini. Stir well until combined.
3. Place the grape seed oil onto a griddle and warm.
4. Pour .25 cup batter on the hot griddle. Leave it along until bubbles begin forming on to surface. Carefully turn over the pancake and cook another four minutes until cooked through.
5. Place the pancakes onto a serving plate and enjoy with some agave syrup.

Nutrition:

- Calories: 246
- Carbohydrates: 49.2 g
- Fiber: 4.6 g
- Protein: 7.8 g

142. Berry Sorbet

Preparation Time: 10 minutes
Cooking Time: 20 minutes
Servings: 6
Ingredients:

- Water, 2 c
- Blend strawberries, 2 c
- Spelt flour, 1.5 tsp.
- Date sugar, .5 c

Directions:

1. Add the water into a large pot and let

the water begin to warm. Add the flour and date sugar and stir until dissolved. Allow this mixture to start boiling and continue to cook for around ten minutes. It should have started to thicken. Take off the heat and set to the side to cool.

2. Once the syrup has cooled off, add in the strawberries, and stir well to combine.
3. Pour into a container that is freezer safe and put it into the freezer until frozen.
4. Take sorbet out of the freezer, cut into chunks, and put it either into a blender or a food processor. Hit the pulse button until the mixture is creamy.
5. Pour this into the same freezer-safe container and put it back into the freezer for four hours.

Nutrition:

- Calories: 99
- Carbohydrates: 8 g

143. Quinoa Porridge

Preparation Time: 5 minutes
Cooking Time: 15 minutes
Servings: 04
Ingredients:

- Zest of one lime
- Coconut milk, .5 c
- Cloves, .5 tsp.
- Ground ginger, 1.5 tsp.
- Spring water, 2 c
- Quinoa, 1 c
- Grated apple, 1

Directions:

1. Cook the quinoa. Follow the instructions on the package. When the quinoa has been cooked, drain well. Place it back into the pot and stir in spices.
2. Add coconut milk and stir well to combine.
3. Grate the apple now and stir well.
4. Divide equally into bowls and add the lime zest on top. Sprinkle with nuts and seeds of choice.

Nutrition:

- Calories: 180
- Fat: 3 g
- Carbohydrates: 40 g
- Protein: 10 g

144. Apple Quinoa

Preparation Time: 15 minutes
Cooking Time: 30 minutes
Servings: 04
Ingredients:

- Coconut oil, 1 tbsp.
- Ginger
- Key lime .5
- Apple, 1
- Quinoa, .5 c
- Optional toppings:
- Seeds
- Nuts
- Berries

Directions:

1. Fix the quinoa according to the instructions on the package. When you are getting close to the end of the cooking time, grate in the apple and cook for 30 seconds.
2. Zest the lime into the quinoa and squeeze the juice in. Stir in the coconut oil.
3. Divide evenly into bowls and sprinkle with some ginger.
4. You can add in some berries, nuts, and seeds right before you eat.

Nutrition:

- Calories: 146
- Fiber: 2.3 g
- Fat: 8.3 g

145. Kamut Porridge

Preparation Time: 10 minutes
Cooking Time: 25 minutes
Servings: 04
Ingredients:

- Agave syrup, 4 tbsp.
- Coconut oil, 1 tbsp.
- Sea salt, .5 tsp.
- Coconut milk, 3.75 c
- Kamut berries, 1 c
- Optional toppings
- Berries
- Coconut chips
- Ground nutmeg
- Ground cloves

Directions:

1. You need to "crack" the Kamut berries. You can try this by placing the berries into a food processor and pulsing until you have 1.25 cups of Kamut.
2. Place the cracked Kamut in a pot with salt and coconut milk. Give it a good stir in order to combine everything. Allow this mixture to come to a full rolling boil and then turn the heat down until the mixture is simmering. Stir every now and then until the Kamut has thickened to your likeness. This normally takes about ten minutes.
3. Take off heat, stir in agave syrup and coconut oil.
4. Garnish with toppings of choice and enjoy.

Nutrition:

- Calories: 114
- Protein: 5 g
- Carbohydrates: 24g
- Fiber: 4 g

146. Hot Kamut with Peaches, Walnuts, and Coconut

Preparation Time: 10 minutes
Cooking Time: 35 minutes
Servings: 04
Ingredients:

- Toasted coconut, 4 tbsp.
- Toasted and chopped walnuts, .5 c
- Chopped dried peaches, 8
- Coconut milk, 3 c
- Kamut cereal, 1 c

Directions:

1. Mix the coconut milk into a saucepan and allow it to warm up. When it begins simmering, add in the Kamut. Let this cook about 15 minutes, while stirring every now and then.
2. When done, divide evenly into bowls and top with the toasted coconut, walnuts, and peaches.
3. You could even go one more and add some fresh berries.

Nutrition:

- Calories: 156
- Protein: 5.8 g
- Carbohydrates: 25 g
- Fiber: 6 g

147. Overnight "Oats"

Preparation Time: 5 minutes
Cooking Time: 0 minutes
Servings: 04
Ingredients:

- Berry of choice, .5 c
- Walnut butter, .5 tbsp.
- Burro banana, .5
- Ginger, .5 tsp.
- Coconut milk, .5 c
- Hemp seeds, .5 c

Directions:

1. Put the hemp seeds, salt, and coconut milk into a glass jar. Mix well.
2. Place the lid on the jar then put it in the refrigerator to sit overnight.
3. The next morning, add the ginger, berries, and banana. Stir well and enjoy it.

Nutrition:

- Calories: 139
- Fat: 4.1 g
- Protein: 9 g
- Sugar: 7 g

148. Blueberry Cupcakes

Preparation Time: 15 minutes
Cooking Time: 40 minutes
Servings: 04
Ingredients:

- Grape seed oil
- Sea salt, .5 tsp.
- Sea moss gel, .25 c
- Agave, .3 c
- Blueberries, .5 c
- Teff flour, .75 c
- Spelt flour, .75 c
- Coconut milk, 1 c

Directions:

1. Warm your oven to 365. Place paper liners into a muffin tin.
2. Place sea moss gel, sea salt, agave, flour, and milk in a large bowl. Mix well to combine. Gently fold in blueberries.
3. Gently pour batter into paper liners. Place in oven and bake 30 minutes.
4. They are done if they have turned a nice golden colour, and they spring back when you touch them.

Nutrition:

- Calories: 85
- Fat: 0.7 g
- Carbohydrates: 12 g
- Protein: 1.4 g
- Fiber: 5 g

149. Brazil Nut Cheese

Preparation Time: 2 hours
Cooking Time: 0 minutes
Servings: 04
Ingredients:

- Grape seed oil, 2 tsp.
- Water, 1.5 c
- Hemp milk, 1.5 c
- Cayenne, .5 tsp.
- Onion powder, 1 tsp.
- Juice of .5 lime
- Sea salt, 2 tsp.
- Brazil nuts, 1 lb.
- Onion powder, 1 tsp.

Directions:

1. You will need to start the process by soaking the Brazil nuts in some water. You just put the nuts into a bowl and make sure the water covers them. Soak no less than two hours or overnight. Overnight would be best.
2. Now you need to put everything except water into a food processor or blender.

3. Add just 5 cups water and blend for two minutes.
4. Continue adding the 5 cups of water and blending until you have the consistency you want.
5. Scrape into an airtight container and enjoy.

Nutrition:

- Calories: 187.
- Protein: 4.1 g
- Fat: 19 g
- Carbs: 3.3 g
- Fiber: 2.1 g

150. Baked Stuffed Pears

Preparation Time: 15 minutes
Cooking Time: 35 minutes
Servings: 04
Ingredients:

- Agave syrup, 4 tbsp.
- Cloves, .25 tsp.
- Chopped walnuts, 4 tbsp.
- Currants, 1 c
- Pears, 4

Directions:

1. Make sure your oven has been warmed to 375.
2. Slice the pears in two lengthwise and remove the core. To get the pear to lay flat, you can slice a small piece off the backside.
3. Place the agave syrup, currants, walnuts, and cloves in a small bowl and mix well. Set this to the side to be used later.
4. Put the pears on a cookie sheet that has parchment paper on it. Make sure the cored sides are facing up. Sprinkle each pear half with about .5 tablespoon of the chopped walnut mixture.
5. Place into the oven and cook for 25 to 30 minutes. Pears should be tender.

Nutrition:

- Calories: 103.9
- Fiber: 3.1 g
- Carbohydrates: 22 g

151. Butternut Squash Pie

Preparation Time: 25 minutes
Cooking Time: 35 minutes
Servings: 04
Ingredients:

For the crust:

- Cold water
- Agave, splash
- Sea salt, a pinch
- Grape seed oil, .5 c
- Coconut flour, .5 c
- Spelt Flour, 1 c

For the filling:

- Butternut squash, peeled, chopped
- Water
- Allspice, to taste
- Agave syrup, to taste
- Hemp milk, 1 c
- Sea moss, 4 tbsp.

Directions:

1. You will need to warm your oven to 350.
2. For the crust:
3. Place the grape seed oil and water into the refrigerator to get it cold. This will take about one hour.
4. Place all ingredients into a large bowl. Now you need to add in the cold water a little bit in small amounts until a dough forms. Place this onto a surface that has been sprinkled with some coconut flour. Knead for a few minutes and roll the dough as thin as you can get it. Carefully, pick it up

and place it inside a pie plate.

5. Place the butternut squash into a Dutch oven and pour in enough water to cover. Bring this to a full rolling boil. Let this cook until the squash has become soft.
6. Completely drain and place into a bowl. Using a potato masher, mash the squash. Add in some allspice and agave to taste. Add in the sea moss and hemp milk. Using a hand mixer, blend well. Pour into the pie crust.
7. Place into an oven and bake for about one hour.

Nutrition:

- Calories: 245
- Carbohydrates: 50 g
- Fat: 10 g

152. Cheesecake

Ingredients:

- Sea salt, .25 tsp.
- Sea moss gel, 1 tbsp.
- Lime juice, 2 tbsp.
- Dates, 5 to 6
- Agave, .25 c
- Hemp or walnut milk, 1.5 c
- Brazil nuts, 2 c

Crust:

- Sea salt, .25 tsp.
- Agave, .25 c
- Coconut flakes, 1.5 c
- Dates, 1.5 c

Topping:

- Blackberries
- Blueberries
- Sliced raspberries
- Sliced strawberry
- Sliced mango

Directions:

1. Mix all of the crust ingredients into your food processor and blend it for about 20 seconds.
2. Spread your crust out into a Springform pan that has been covered with parchment.
3. Place the mango slices along the side of the pan and then place it in the freezer as you prepare everything else.
4. Add everything for the cheesecake to your blender and mix it until it creates a smooth mixture.
5. Get rid of the Springform pan from the freezer and pour the filling in. Wrap in foil and let it sit for three to four hours.
6. Carefully remove from the pan, and then place the rest of the toppings over the top. All of the leftovers should be kept in the freezer.

153. Coconut Chia Cream Pot

Preparation Time: 5 minutes

Cooking Time: 5 minutes

Servings: 04

Ingredients:

- Date, one (1)
- Coconut milk (organic), one (1) cup
- Coconut yogurt, one (1) cup
- Vanilla extract, ½ teaspoon
- Chia seeds, ¼ cup
- Sesame seeds, one (1) teaspoon
- Flaxseed (ground), one (1) tablespoon or flax meal, one (1) tablespoon

Toppings:

- Fig, one (1)
- Blueberries, one (1) handful
- Mixed nuts (brazil nuts, almonds, pistachios, macadamia, etc.)
- Cinnamon (ground), one teaspoon

Directions:

1. First, blend the date with coconut milk (the idea is to sweeten the coconut milk).
2. Get a mixing bowl and add the coconut milk with the vanilla, sesame seeds, chia seeds, and flax meal.
3. Refrigerate for between twenty to thirty minutes or wait till the chia expands.
4. To serve, pour a layer of coconut yogurt in a small glass, then add the chia mix, followed by pouring another layer of the coconut yogurt.
5. It's alkaline, creamy, and delicious.

Nutrition:

- Calories: 310
- Carbohydrates: 39 g
- Protein: 4 g
- Fiber: 8.1 g

154. Chocolate Avocado Mousse

Preparation Time: 10 minutes
Cooking Time: 5 minutes
Servings: 04
Ingredients:

- Coconut water, 2/3 cup
- Hass avocado, ½
- Raw cacao, 2 teaspoons
- Vanilla, 1 teaspoon
- Dates, three (3)
- Sea salt, one (1) teaspoon
- Dark chocolate shavings

Directions:

1. Blend all ingredients.
2. Blast until it becomes thick and smooth, as you wish.
3. Put in a fridge and allow it to get firm.

Nutrition:

- Calories: 181.8
- Fat: 151. g
- Protein: 12 g

155. Chia Vanilla Coconut Pudding

Preparation Time: 5 minutes
Cooking Time: 5 minutes
Servings: 2
Ingredients:

- Coconut oil, 2 tablespoons
- Raw cashew, ½ cup
- Coconut water, ½ cup
- Cinnamon, 1 teaspoon
- Dates (pitted), 3
- Vanilla, 2 teaspoons
- Coconut flakes (unsweetened), 1 teaspoon
- Salt (Himalayan or Celtic Grey)
- Chia seeds, 6 tablespoons
- Cinnamon or pomegranate seeds for garnish (optional)

Directions:

1. Get a blender, add all the ingredients (minus the pomegranate and chia seeds), and blend for about forty to sixty seconds.
2. Reduce the blender speed to the lowest and add the chia seeds.
3. Pour the content into an airtight container and put it in a refrigerator for five to six hours.
4. To serve, you can garnish with the cinnamon powder of pomegranate seeds.

Nutrition:

- Calories: 201
- Fat: 10 g
- Sodium: 32.8 mg

156. Sweet Tahini Dip with Ginger Cinnamon Fruit

Preparation Time: 10 minutes
Cooking Time: 5 minutes
Servings: 2
Ingredients:

- Cinnamon, one (1) teaspoon
- Green apple, one (1)
- Pear, one (1)
- Fresh ginger, two (2) or three (3)
- Celtic sea salt, one (1) teaspoon

Ingredients for sweet Tahini:

- Almond butter (raw), three (3) teaspoons
- Tahini (one big scoop), three (3) teaspoons
- Coconut oil, two (2) teaspoons
- Cayenne (optional), ¼ teaspoons
- Wheat-free tamari, two (2) teaspoons
- Liquid coconut nectar, one (1) teaspoon

Directions:

1. Get a clean mixing bowl.
2. Grate the ginger, add cinnamon, sea salt, and mix in the bowl.
3. Dice apple and pear into little cubes, turn into the bowl, and mix.
4. Get a mixing bowl and mix all the ingredients.
5. Then, add the sprinkle, the sweet Tahini, and dip all over the ginger cinnamon fruit.
6. Serve.

Nutrition:

- Calories: 109
- Fat: 10.8 g
- Sodium: 258 mg

157. Coconut Butter and Chopped Berries with Mint

Preparation Time: 5 minutes
Cooking Time: 5 minutes
Servings: 04
Ingredients:

- Chopped mint, one (1) tablespoon
- Coconut butter (melted), two (2) tablespoons
- Mixed berries (strawberries, blueberries, and raspberries)

Directions:

1. Get a small bowl and add the berries.
2. Drizzle the melted coconut butter and sprinkle the mint.
3. Serve.

Nutrition:

- Calories: 159
- Fat: 12 g
- Carbohydrates: 18 g

158. Alkaline Raw Pumpkin Pie

Preparation Time: 5 minutes
Cooking Time: 5 minutes
Servings: 04
Ingredients:

Ingredients for pie crust:

- Cinnamon, one (1) teaspoon
- Dates/Turkish apricots, one (1) cup
- Raw almonds, one (1) cup
- Coconut flakes (unsweetened), one (1) cup

Ingredients for pie filling:

- Dates, six (6)
- Cinnamon, ½ teaspoon
- Nutmeg, ½ teaspoon
- Pecans (soaked overnight), one (1) cup
- Organic pumpkin Blends (12 oz.), 1 ¼ cup

- Nutmeg, ½ teaspoon
- Sea salt (Himalayan or Celtic Sea Salt), ¼ teaspoon
- Vanilla, 1 teaspoon
- Gluten-free tamari

Directions:

Directions for pie crust:

1. Get a food processor and blend all the pie crust ingredients at the same time.
2. Make sure the mixture turns oily and sticky before you stop mixing.
3. Put the mixture in a pie pan and mold against the sides and floor, to make it stick properly.

Directions for the pie filling:

1. Mix ingredients together in a blender.
2. Add the mixture to fill in the pie crust.
3. Pour some cinnamon on top.
4. Refrigerate until it's cold and then mold.

Nutrition:

- Calories 135
- Calories from Fat 41.4.
- Total Fat 4.6 g
- Cholesterol 11.3 mg

159. Strawberry Sorbet

Preparation Time: 5 minutes
Cooking Time: 4 hours
Servings: 4
Ingredients:

- 2 cups of strawberries*
- 1 1/2 teaspoons of spelt flour
- 1/2 cup of date sugar
- 2 cups of spring water

Directions:

1. Add date sugar, spring water, and spelt flour to a medium pot and boil on low heat for about ten minutes. The mixture should thicken, like syrup.
2. Remove the pot from the heat and allow it to cool.
3. After cooling, add Blend Strawberry and mix gently.
4. Put the mixture in a container and freeze.
5. Cut it into pieces, put the sorbet into a processor, and blend until smooth.
6. Put everything back in the container and leave in the refrigerator for at least four hours.
7. Serve and enjoy your Strawberry Sorbet!

Nutrition:

- Calories: 198
- Carbohydrates: 28 g

160. Blueberry Muffins

Preparation Time: 5 minutes
Cooking Time: 1 Hour
Servings: 3
Ingredients:

- 1/2 cup of blueberries
- 3/4 cup of teff flour
- 3/4 cup of spelt flour
- 1/3 cup of agave syrup
- 1/2 teaspoon of pure sea salt
- 1 cup of coconut milk
- 1/4 cup of sea moss gel (optional, check information)
- Grape Seed Oil

Directions:

1. Preheat your oven to 365 degrees Fahrenheit.
2. Grease or line 6 standard muffin cups.
3. Add Teff, Spelt flour, Pure Sea Salt, Coconut Milk, Sea Moss Gel, and Agave Syrup to a large bowl. Mix

them together.
4. Add Blueberries to the mixture and mix well.
5. Divide muffin batter among the 6 muffin cups.
6. Bake for 30 minutes until golden brown.
7. Serve and enjoy your Blueberry Muffins!

Nutrition:

- Calories: 65
- Fat: 0.7 g
- Carbohydrates: 12 g
- Protein: 1.4 g
- Fiber: 5 g

161. Banana Strawberry Ice Cream

Preparation Time: 5 minutes
Cooking Time: 4 hours
Servings: 5
Ingredients:

- 1 cup of strawberry*
- 5 quartered baby bananas*
- 1/2 avocado, chopped
- 1 tablespoon of agave syrup
- 1/4 cup of homemade walnut milk

Directions:

1. Mix ingredients into the blender and blend them well.
2. Taste. If it is too thick, add extra milk or agave syrup if you want it sweeter.
3. Put in a container with a lid and allow to freeze for at least 5 to 6 hours.
4. Serve it and enjoy your banana strawberry ice cream!

Nutrition:

- Calories: 200
- Fat: 0.5 g
- Carbohydrates: 44 g

162. Homemade Whipped Cream

Preparation Time: 5 minutes
Cooking Time: 10 minutes
Servings: 1 Cup
Ingredients:

- 1 cup of Aquafaba
- 1/4 cup of agave syrup

Directions:

1. Add agave syrup and Aquafaba into a bowl.
2. Mix at high speed around 5 minutes with a stand mixer or 10 to 15 minutes with a hand mixer.
3. Serve and enjoy your homemade whipped cream!

Nutrition:

- Calories: 21
- Fat: 0g
- Sodium: 0.3g
- Carbohydrates: 5.3g
- Fiber: 0g
- Sugars: 4.7g
- Protein: 0g

163. "Chocolate" Pudding

Preparation Time: 5 minutes
Cooking Time: 20 minutes
Servings: 4
Ingredients:

- 1 to 2 cups of black sapote
- 1/4 cup of agave syrup
- 1/2 cup of soaked Brazil nuts (overnight or for at least 3 hours)
- 1 tablespoon of hemp seeds
- 1/2 cup of spring water

Directions:

1. Cut 1 to 2 cups of black sapote in half.
2. Remove all seeds. You should have 1 full cup of de-seeded fruit.
3. Mix all ingredients into a blender and

blend until smooth.
4. Serve and enjoy your "chocolate" pudding!

Nutrition:

- Calories: 134
- Fat: 0.5 g
- Carbohydrates: 15 g
- Protein: 2.5 g
- Fiber: 10 g

164. Banana Nut Muffins

Preparation Time: 5 minutes
Cooking Time: 1 Hour
Servings: 6
Ingredients:
Dry ingredients:

- 1 1/2 cups of spelt or teff flour
- 1/2 teaspoon of pure sea salt
- 3/4 cup of date syrup

Wet ingredients:

- 2 medium blended burro bananas
- ¼ cup of grape seed oil
- ¾ cup of homemade walnut milk (see recipe)*
- 1 tablespoon of key lime juice

Filling ingredients:

- ½ cup of chopped walnuts (plus extra for decorating)
- 1 chopped burro banana

Directions:

1. Preheat your oven to 400 degrees Fahrenheit.
2. Take a muffin tray and grease 12 cups or line with cupcake liners.
3. Put all dry ingredients in a large bowl and mix them thoroughly.
4. Add all wet ingredients to a separate, smaller bowl and mix well with blended bananas.
5. Mix ingredients from the two bowls in one large container. Be careful not to over mix.
6. Add the filling ingredients and fold in gently.
7. Pour muffin batter into the 12 prepared muffin cups and garnish with a couple of Walnuts.
8. Bake it for 22 to 26 minutes until golden brown.
9. Allow cooling for 10 minutes.
10. Serve and enjoy your banana nut muffins!

Nutrition:

- Calories: 150
- Fat: 10 g
- Carbohydrates: 30 g
- Protein: 2.4 g
- Fiber: 2 g

165. Mango Nut Cheesecake

Cooking Time: 4 Hour 30 Minutes
Servings: 8 Servings
Ingredients:
Filling:

- 2 cups of Brazil nuts
- 5 to 6 dates
- 1 tablespoon of sea moss gel (check information)
- 1/4 cup of agave syrup
- 1/4 teaspoon of pure sea salt
- 2 tablespoons of lime juice
- 1 1/2 cups of homemade walnut milk (see recipe)*

Crust:

- 1 1/2 cups of quartered dates
- 1/4 cup of agave syrup
- 1 1/2 cups of coconut flakes
- 1/4 teaspoon of pure sea salt

Toppings:

- Sliced mango
- Sliced strawberries

Directions:

- Put all crust ingredients in a food processor and blend for 30 seconds.
- With parchment paper, cover a baking form and spread out the blended crust ingredients.
- Put sliced mango across the crust and freeze for 10 minutes.
- Mix all filling ingredients using a blender until it becomes smooth.
- Pour the filling above the crust, cover with foil or parchment paper, and let it stand for about 3 to 4 hours in the refrigerator.
- Take out from the baking form and garnish with toppings.
- Serve and enjoy your mango nut cheesecake!

166. Blackberry Jam

Preparation Time: 5 minutes
Cooking Time: 4 hours 30 minutes
Servings: 1 cup
Ingredients:

- 3/4 cup of blackberries
- 1 tablespoon of key lime juice
- 3 tablespoons of agave syrup
- ¼ cup of sea moss gel + extra 2 tablespoons (check information)

Directions:

1. Put rinsed blackberries into a medium pot and cook on medium heat.
2. Stir blackberries until liquid appears.
3. Once berries soften, use your immersion blender to chop up any large pieces. If you don't have a blender put the mixture in a food processor, mix it well, then return to the pot.
4. Add sea moss gel, key lime juice, and agave syrup to the blended mixture. Boil on medium heat and stir well until it becomes thick.
5. Remove from the heat and leave it to cool for 10 minutes.
6. Serve it with bread pieces or the Flatbread (see recipe).
7. Enjoy your blackberry jam!

Nutrition:

- Calories: 43
- Fat: 0.5 g
- Carbohydrates: 13 g

167. Blackberry Bars

Preparation Time: 5 minutes
Cooking Time: 1 hour 20 minutes
Servings: 4
Ingredients:

- 3 burro bananas or 4 baby bananas
- 1 cup of spelt flour
- 2 cups of quinoa flakes
- 1/4 cup of agave syrup
- 1/4 teaspoon of pure sea salt
- 1/2 cup of grape seed oil
- 1 cup of prepared blackberry jam

Directions:

1. Preheat your oven to 350 degrees Fahrenheit.
2. Remove the skin of the bananas and mash with a fork in a large bowl.
3. Combine agave syrup and grape seed oil with the blend and mix well.
4. Add spelt flour and quinoa flakes. Knead the dough until it becomes sticky to your fingers.
5. Cover a 9x9-inch baking pan with parchment paper.
6. Take 2/3 of the dough and smooth it out over the parchment pan with your fingers.
7. Spread blackberry jam over the

dough.

8. Crumble the remaining dough and sprinkle on the top.
9. Bake for 20 minutes.
10. Remove from the oven and let it cool for at 10 to 15 minutes.
11. Cut into small pieces.
12. Serve and enjoy your blackberry bars!

Nutrition:

- Calories: 43
- Fat: 0.5 g
- Carbohydrates: 10 g
- Protein: 1.4 g
- Fiber: 5 g

Chapter 10: Smoothies

168. Raisins – Plume Smoothie (RPS)

Preparation Time: 10 minutes
Cooking Time: 0 minutes
Servings: 1
Ingredients:

- 1 teaspoon raisins
- 2 sweet cherry
- 1 skinned black plume
- 1 cup Dr. Sebi's stomach calming herbal tea/cuachalalate back powder
- ¼ coconut water

Directions:

1. Flash 1 teaspoon of raisins in warm water for 5 seconds and drain the water completely.
2. Rinse, cube sweet cherry and skinned black plum
3. Get 1 cup of water boiled; put ¾ Dr. Sebi's stomach calming herbal tea for 10 – 15minutes.
4. If you are unable to get Dr. Sebi's stomach calming herbal tea, you can alternatively cook 1 teaspoon of powdered cuachalalate with 1 cup of water for 5 – 10 minutes, remove the extract and allow it to cool.
5. Pour all the ARPS items inside a blender and blend till you achieve a homogenous smoothie.
6. It is now okay for you to enjoy the inevitable detox smoothie.

Nutrition:

- Calories: 150
- Fat: 1.2 g
- Carbohydrates: 79 g
- Protein: 3.1 g

169. Nori Clove Smoothies (NCS)

Preparation Time: 10 minutes
Cooking Time: 0 minutes
Servings: 1
Ingredients:

- ¼ cup fresh nori
- 1 cup cubed banana
- 1 teaspoon diced onion or ¼ teaspoon powdered onion
- ½ teaspoon clove
- 1 cup Dr. Sebi's energy booster
- 1 tablespoon agave syrup

Directions:

1. Rinse ANCS Items with clean water.
2. Finely chop the onion to take one teaspoon and cut fresh nori.
3. Boil 1½ teaspoon with 2 cups of water, remove the particle, allow to cool, measure 1 cup of the tea extract.
4. Pour all the items inside a blender with the tea extract and blend to achieve homogenous smoothies.
5. Transfer into a clean cup and have a nice time with a lovely body detox and energizer.

Nutrition:

- Calories: 78
- Fat: 2.3 g
- Carbohydrates: 5 g
- Protein: 6 g

170. Brazil Lettuce Smoothies (BLS)

Preparation Time: 10 minutes
Cooking Time: 0 minutes
Servings: 1
Ingredients:

- 1 cup raspberries
- ½ handful Romaine lettuce
- ½ cup homemade walnut milk
- 2 Brazil nuts
- ½ large grape with seed
- 1 cup soft jelly coconut water
- Date Sugar to Taste

Directions:

1. In a clean bowl rinse the fruits with clean water.
2. Chop the Romaine lettuce and cubed raspberries and add other items into the blender and blend to achieve homogenous smoothies.
3. Serve your delicious medicinal detox.

Nutrition:

- Calories: 168
- Fat: 4.5 g
- Carbohydrates: 31.3 g
- Sugar: 19.2 g
- Protein: 3.6 g

171. Apple – Banana Smoothie (ABS)

Preparation Time: 10 minutes
Cooking Time: 0 minutes
Servings: 1
Ingredients:

- 1 cup cubed apple
- ½ burro banana
- ½ cup cubed mango
- ½ cup cubed watermelon
- ½ teaspoon powdered onion
- 3 tablespoon Key lime juice
- Date sugar to taste (If you like)

Directions:

1. In a clean bowl rinse the fruits with clean water.
2. Add cubed banana, apple, mango, watermelon, and add other items into the blender and blend to achieve homogenous smoothies.
3. Serve your delicious medicinal detox.
4. Alternatively, you can add one tablespoon of finely dices raw red onion if the powdered onion is not available.

Nutrition:

- Calories: 99
- Fat: 0.3g
- Carbohydrates: 23 grams
- Protein: 1.1 g

172. Ginger – Pear Smoothie (GPS)

Preparation Time: 10 minutes
Cooking Time: 0 minutes
Servings: 1
Ingredients:

- 1 big pear with seed and cured
- ½ avocado
- ¼ handful watercress
- ½ sour orange
- ½ cup of ginger tea
- ½ cup of coconut water
- ¼ cup of spring water
- 2 tablespoons agave syrup
- Date sugar to satisfaction

Directions:

1. Firstly, boil 1 cup of ginger tea, cover the cup and allow it cool to room temperature.
2. Pour all the AGPS Items into your clean blender and homogenize them

to smooth fluid.

3. You have just prepared yourself a wonderful detox Romaine smoothie.

Nutrition:

- Calories: 101.
- Protein: 1 g
- Carbs: 27 g
- Fiber: 6 g

173. Cantaloupe – Amaranth Smoothie (CAS)

Preparation Time: 10 minutes
Cooking Time: 0 minutes
Servings: 1
Ingredients:

- ½ cup of cubed cantaloupe
- ¼ handful green amaranth
- ½ cup homemade hemp milk
- ¼ teaspoon Dr. Sebi's bromide plus powder
- 1 cup of coconut water
- 1 teaspoon agave syrup

Directions:

1. You will have to rinse all the ACAS items with clean water.
2. Chop green amaranth, cubed cantaloupe, transfer all into a blender and blend to achieve a homogenous smoothie.
3. Pour into a clean cup; add Agave syrup and homemade hemp milk.
4. Stir them together and drink.

Nutrition:

- Calories: 55
- Fiber: 1.5 g
- Carbohydrates: 8 mg

174. Garbanzo Squash Smoothie (GSS)

Preparation Time: 10 minutes
Cooking Time: 0 minutes
Servings: 1
Ingredients:

- 1 large cubed apple
- 1 fresh tomato
- 1 tablespoon finely chopped fresh onion or ¼ teaspoon powdered onion
- ¼ cup boiled garbanzo bean
- ½ cup of coconut milk
- ¼ cubed Mexican squash chayote
- 1 cup energy booster tea

Directions:

1. You will need to rinse the AGSS items with clean water.
2. Boil 1½ Dr. Sebi's energy booster tea with 2 cups of clean water. Filter the extract, measure 1 cup, and allow it to cool.
3. Cook Garbanzo beans, drain the water and allow it to cool.
4. Pour all the AGSS items into a high-speed blender and blend to achieve a homogenous smoothie.
5. You may add date sugar.
6. Serve your amazing smoothie and drink.

Nutrition:

- Calories: 82.
- Carbs: 22 g
- Protein: 2 g
- Fiber: 7 g

175. Strawberry – Orange Smoothies (SOS)

Preparation Time: 10 minutes
Cooking Time: 0 minutes
Servings: 1
Ingredients:

- 1 cup of diced strawberries
- 1 removed back of Seville orange
- ¼ cup cubed cucumber
- ¼ cup Romaine lettuce
- ½ kelp
- ½ burro banana
- 1 cup soft jelly coconut water
- ½ cup of water
- Date sugar.

Directions:

1. Use clean water to rinse all the vegetable items of ASOS into a clean bowl.
2. Chop Romaine lettuce; dice strawberry, cucumber, and banana; remove the back of Seville orange and divide into four.
3. Transfer all the ASOS items inside a clean blender and blend to achieve a homogenous smoothie.
4. Pour into a clean big cup and fortify your body with a palatable detox.

Nutrition:

- Calories 298
- Calories from Fat 9.
- Fat 1g
- Cholesterol 2mg
- Sodium 73mg
- Potassium 998mg
- Carbohydrates 68g
- Fiber 7g
- Sugar 50g

176. Tamarind – Pear Smoothie (TPS)

Preparation Time: 10 minutes
Cooking Time: 0 minutes
Servings: 1
Ingredients:

- ½ burro banana
- ½ cup of watermelon
- 1 raspberry
- 1 prickly pear
- 1 grape with seed
- 3 tamarinds
- ½ medium cucumber
- 1 cup of coconut water
- ½ cup Distilled water

Directions:

1. Use clean water to rinse all the ATPS items.
2. Remove the pod of tamarinds and collect the edible part around the seed into a container.
3. If you must use the seeds, then you have to boil the seed for 15 minutes and add to the tamarind edible part in the container.
4. Cube all other vegetable fruits and transfer all the items into a high-speed blender and blend to achieve a homogenous smoothie.

Nutrition:

- Calories: 199
- Carbohydrates: 47 g
- Fat: 1g
- Protein: 6g

177. Currant Elderberry Smoothie (CES)

Preparation Time: 10 minutes
Cooking Time: 0 minutes
Servings: 1
Ingredients:

- ¼ cup cubed elderberry
- 1 sour cherry
- 2 currants
- 1 cubed burro banana
- 1 fig
- 1 cup 4 bay leaves tea
- 1 cup energy booster tea
- Date sugar to your satisfaction

Directions:

1. Use clean water to rinse all the ACES items.
2. Initially boil ¾ teaspoon of energy Booster Tea with 2 cups of water on a heat source and allow boiling for 10 minutes.
3. Add 4 bay leaves and boil together for another 4 minutes.
4. Drain the tea extract into a clean big cup and allow it to cool.
5. Transfer all the items into a high-speed blender and blend till you achieve a homogenous smoothie.
6. Pour the palatable medicinal smoothie into a clean cup and drink.

Nutrition:

- Calories: 63
- Fat: 0.22g
- Sodium: 1.1mg
- Carbohydrates: 15.5g
- Fiber: 4.8g
- Sugars: 8.25g
- Protein: 1.6g

178. Sweet Dream Strawberry Smoothie

Preparation Time: 15 minutes
Cooking Time: 0
Servings: 1
Ingredients:

- 5 strawberries
- 3 dates – pits eliminated
- 2 burro bananas or small bananas
- Spring water for 32 fluid ounce of smoothie

Directions:

1. Strip off the skin of the bananas.
2. Wash the dates and strawberries.
3. Include bananas, dates, and strawberries to a blender container.
4. Include a couple of water and blend.
5. Keep on including adequate water to persuade up to be 32 oz. of smoothie.

Nutrition:

- Calories: 282
- Fat: 11g
- Carbohydrates: 4g
- Protein: 7g

179. Alkaline Green Ginger and Banana Cleansing Smoothie

Preparation Time: 15 minutes
Cooking Time: 0
Servings: 1
Ingredients:

- One handful of kale
- One banana, frozen
- Two cups of hemp seed milk
- One inch of ginger, finely minced
- Half cup of chopped strawberries, frozen
- 1 tablespoon of agave or your preferred sweetener

Directions:

1. Mix all the ingredients in a blender and mix on high speed.
2. Allow it to blend evenly.
3. Pour into a pitcher with a few decorative straws and voila, you are one happy camper.
4. Enjoy!

Nutrition:

- Calories: 350
- Fat: 4g
- Carbohydrates: 52g
- Protein: 16g

180. Orange Mixed Detox Smoothie

Preparation Time: 15 minutes
Cooking Time: 0
Servings: 1
Ingredients:

- One cup of veggies (amaranth, dandelion, lettuce or watercress)
- Half avocado
- One cup of tender-jelly coconut water
- One Seville orange
- Juice of one key lime
- One tablespoon of bromide plus powder

Directions:

1. Peel and cut the Seville orange in chunks.
2. Mix all the ingredients collectively in a high-speed blender until done.

Nutrition:

- Calories: 71
- Fat: 1g
- Carbohydrates: 12g
- Protein: 2g

181. Cucumber Toxin Flush Smoothie

Preparation Time: 15 minutes
Cooking Time: 0
Servings: 1
Ingredients:

- 1 cucumber
- 1 key lime
- 1 cup of watermelon (seeded), cubed

Directions:

1. Mix all the above ingredients in a high-speed blender.
2. Considering that watermelon and cucumbers are largely water, you may not want to add any extra, however, you can do so if you want.
3. Juice the key lime and add it to your smoothie.
4. Enjoy!

Nutrition:

- Calories: 219
- Fat: 4g
- Carbohydrates: 48g
- Protein: 5g

182. Apple Blueberry Smoothie

Preparation Time: 15 minutes
Cooking Time: 0
Servings: 1
Ingredients:

- Half apple
- One date
- Half cup of blueberries
- Half cup of sparkling callaloo
- One tablespoon of hemp seeds
- One tablespoon of sesame seeds
- Two cups of sparkling soft-jelly coconut water
- Half tablespoon of bromide plus powder

Directions:

1. Mix all of the ingredients in a high-speed blender and enjoy!

Nutrition:

- Calories: 167.4
- Fat: 6.4g
- Carbohydrates: 22.5g
- Protein: 6.7g

183. Detox Berry Smoothie

Preparation Time: 15 minutes
Cooking Time: 0
Servings: 1
Ingredients:

- Spring water
- 1/4 avocado, pitted
- One medium burro banana
- One Seville orange
- Two cups of fresh lettuce
- One tablespoon of hemp seeds
- One cup of berries (blueberries or an aggregate of blueberries, strawberries, and raspberries)

Directions:

1. Add the spring water to your blender.
2. Put the fruits and veggies right inside the blender.
3. Blend all ingredients until smooth.

Nutrition:

- Calories: 202.4
- Fat: 4.5g
- Carbohydrates: 32.9g
- Protein: 13.3g

184. Papaya Detox Smoothie

Preparation Time: 15 minutes
Cooking Time: 0
Servings: 1
Ingredients:

- Two cups papaya
- One tablespoon of papaya seeds
- Juice of a Lime
- One cup of filtered water

Directions:

1. Chop the papaya into square portions and scoop out a tablespoon of clean and raw papaya seeds.
2. Mix all of the ingredients right into a high-speed blender for 1 minute until the whole thing is blended.
3. Pour into a tumbler and enjoy this tasty drink your liver will love.
4. Enjoy!

Nutrition:

- Calories: 197
- Fat: 0.7g
- Carbohydrates: 49.4g
- Protein: 5.4g

185. Apple and Amaranth Detoxifying Smoothie

Preparation Time: 15 minutes
Cooking Time: 0
Servings: 1
Ingredients:

- 1/4 avocado
- 1 key lime
- Two apples, chopped
- Two cups of water
- Two cups of amaranth veggie

Directions:

1. Put all the ingredients collectively in a blender.
2. Blend all the ingredients evenly.
3. Enjoy this delicious smoothie.

Nutrition:

- Calories: 133
- Fat: 4g
- Carbohydrates: 24g
- Protein: 3g

186. Avocado Mixed Smoothie

Preparation Time: 15 minutes
Cooking Time: 0
Servings: 1
Ingredients:

- One cup of water
- One ounce of blueberries
- One pear, chopped
- 1/4 avocado, pitted
- 1/4 cup cooked quinoa

Directions:

1. Mix all ingredients in a high-speed blender and enjoy!

Nutrition:

- Calories: 187
- Fat: 21g
- Carbohydrates: 29g
- Protein: 11g

187. Peach Berry Smoothie

Preparation Time: 15 minutes
Cooking Time: 0
Servings: 1
Ingredients:

- Half cup of frozen peaches
- Half cup of frozen blueberries
- Half cup of frozen cherries
- Half cup of frozen strawberries
- One tablespoon of sea moss gel
- One tablespoon of hemp seeds
- One tablespoon of coconut water
- One tablespoon of agave

Directions:

1. Blend all ingredients for one minute.
2. If the combination is too thick, add extra ¼ cup of coconut water and blend for another 20 secs.
3. Enjoy your peach berry smoothie!

Nutrition:

- Calories: 170
- Fat: 0g
- Carbohydrates: 43g
- Protein: 0g

188. Irish Sea Moss Smoothie

Preparation Time: 15 minutes
Cooking Time: 0
Servings: 1
Ingredients:

- 2 oz. of whole wild sea moss, soaked
- 2 cups of spring water

Directions:

1. To prepare Irish sea moss smoothie, use two whole and wild sea moss.
2. Carefully wash away any sand and debris.
3. Do a final wash and chop up longer ones to safeguard your blender's blade.
4. Add your sea moss and two cups of spring water to blend in the blender.
5. Put in a jar and refrigerate. This smoothie can last for many weeks.
6. Enjoy your delicious smoothie.

Nutrition:

- Calories: 220
- Fat: 3g
- Carbohydrates: 45g
- Protein: 2g

189. Cucumber Mixed Detox Smoothie

Preparation Time: 15 minutes
Cooking Time: 0
Servings: 1
Ingredients:

- Half cucumber, chopped
- One inch of ginger
- One pinch of pure sea salt
- Two grapefruits, squeezed

- Two lemons, squeezed
- One avocado, chopped
- Half cup of filtered or spring water
- One pinch cayenne pepper

Directions:

1. Blend all ingredients. Sip and experience this tasty nutritious smoothie!

Nutrition:

- Calories: 48
- Fat: 0g
- Carbohydrates: 12g
- Protein: 1g

190. Strawberry Banana Smoothie

Preparation Time: 15 minutes
Cooking Time: 0
Servings: 1-2
Ingredients:

- 2 cups hemp milk
- 4 banana
- 8 oz. strawberry
- ¾ cup dates
- 1 tbsp. agave

Directions:

1. To make this delicious smoothie, you need to place the strawberries and date in a high-speed blender.
2. Blend them for a minute or two or until they are slightly broken down.
3. After that, add the banana along with the hemp milk and agave.
4. Blend them for 2 to 3 minutes or until combined well.
5. Enjoy.

Nutrition:

- Calories: 148
- Fat: 2g
- Carbohydrates: 21g
- Protein: 1g

191. Green Monster Smoothie

Preparation Time: 15 minutes
Cooking Time: 0
Servings: 1
Ingredients:

- ½ of 1 avocado, diced
- ½ of 1 mango, diced
- 2 to 3 dates, pitted
- 1 tbsp. soursop pulp
- 1 bunch of rainbow Kale, leaves torn
- ½ cup of coconut water

Directions:

1. To make this smoothie, place all the ingredients in a high-speed blender and blend it for 2 to 3 minutes or until everything comes together and smooth.
2. Move the mixture to a serving glass and serve it with ice cubes if you desire to take it cold.

Nutrition:

- Calories: 179.4
- Fat: 2.3g
- Carbohydrates: 36.8g
- Protein: 6.8g

192. Apple Smoothie

Preparation Time: 15 minutes
Cooking Time: 0
Servings: 2
Ingredients:

- 2 cups of apple juice, fresh
- 2 cups ice cube
- 1 tbsp. sea moss
- 1 clove, grounded
- 1 tbsp. ginger, grounded

Directions:

1. To start with, place all the ingredients needed to make the smoothie in a high-speed blender. Blend all

ingredients wait for 2 to 3 minutes or until you get a smooth mixture.

2. Serve and enjoy.

Nutrition:

- Calories: 431.5
- Fat: 10.8g
- Carbohydrates: 53.1g
- Protein: 38.4g

193. Weight Loss Apple Cucumber Smoothie

Preparation Time: 15 minutes

Cooking Time: 0

Servings: 1

Ingredients:

- One large to medium size of sliced cucumber
- One large cubed apple
- One large sliced bell pepper
- Six seeded dates (rinsed)
- Six large strawberries
- Five sliced tomatoes (rinsed)
- Half to one cupful of water

Directions:

1. Combine the whole recipes and blend very well until smooth. Wow! The first-day breakfast is settled, enjoy.

Nutrition:

- 65 calories
- Carb 57 g
- Protein 2 g
- Fat 4 g

194. Toxins Removal Smoothie

Preparation Time: 15 minutes

Cooking Time: 0

Servings: 1

Ingredients:

- One seeded and sliced small to large-sized watermelon
- One large key lime (removes the juice and discards the seed
- One large cucumber (sliced)

Directions:

1. Transfer the lime juice into the blender.
2. Add the remaining recipes and blend very well to obtain a smooth mixture.
3. Wow! This means you have successfully completed the second-day smoothie. Enjoy.

Nutrition:

- 45 calories
- Carb 35 g
- Protein 6 g
- Fat 4 g

195. Multiple Berries Smoothie

Preparation Time: 15 minutes

Cooking Time: 0

Servings: 1

Ingredients:

- A quarter cupful of blueberries
- A quarter cupful of strawberries
- A quarter cupful of raspberries
- One large banana (peeled and sliced)
- Agave syrup as desired
- A half cupful of water

Directions:

1. Transfer the water into the blender.
2. Add the remaining recipes and blend until smooth.
3. I really love this smoothie because it is very sweet without adding sugar and the colour is also inviting.

Nutrition:

- Calories: 210
- Carbohydrates: 55 g
- Sodium: 20 mg

196. Dandelion Avocado Smoothie

Preparation Time: 15 minutes
Cooking Time: 0
Servings: 1
Ingredients:

- One cup of dandelion
- One orange (juiced)
- Coconut water
- One avocado
- One key lime (juice)

Directions:

1. In a high-speed blend all ingredients until smooth.

Nutrition:

- Calories: 160
- Fat: 15 grams
- Carbohydrates: 9 grams
- Protein: 2 grams

197. Amaranth Greens and Avocado Smoothie

Preparation Time: 15 minutes
Cooking Time: 0
Servings: 1
Ingredients:

- One key lime (juice)
- Two sliced apples (seeded)
- Half avocado
- Two cups of amaranth greens
- Two cups of watercress
- One cup of water

Directions:

1. Add the whole recipes together and transfer them into the blender. Blend thoroughly until smooth.

Nutrition:

- Calories: 160
- Fat: 15 grams
- Carbohydrates: 9 grams
- Protein: 2 grams

198. Lettuce, Orange and Banana Smoothie

Preparation Time: 15 minutes
Cooking Time: 0
Servings: 1
Ingredients:

- One and a half cupsful of fresh lettuce
- One large banana
- One cup of mixed berries of your choice
- One juiced orange

Directions:

1. First, add the orange juice to your blender.
2. Add the remaining recipes and blend thoroughly.
3. Enjoy the rest of your day.

Nutrition:

- Calories: 252.1
- Protein: 4.1 g

199. Delicious Elderberry Smoothie

Preparation Time: 15 minutes
Cooking Time: 0
Servings: 1
Ingredients:

- One cupful of elderberry
- One cupful of cucumber
- One large apple
- A quarter cupful of water

Directions:

1. Add the whole recipes together into a blender. Grind very well until they are uniformly smooth and enjoy.

Nutrition:

- Calories: 106
- Carbohydrates: 26.68

200. Peaches Zucchini Smoothie

Preparation Time: 15 minutes
Cooking Time: 0
Servings: 1
Ingredients:

- A half cupful of squash
- A half cupful of peaches
- A quarter cupful of coconut water
- A half cupful of Zucchini

Directions:

1. Add the whole recipes together into a blender and blend until smooth and serve.

Nutrition:

- 55 Calories
- 0g Fat
- 2g Protein
- 10mg Sodium
- 14g Carbohydrate
- 2g Fiber

201. Ginger Orange and Strawberry Smoothie

Preparation Time: 15 minutes
Cooking Time: 0
Servings: 1
Ingredients:

- One cup of strawberry
- One large orange (juice)
- One large banana
- Quarter small sized ginger (peeled and sliced)

Directions:

1. Transfer the orange juice to a clean blender.
2. Add the remaining recipes and blend thoroughly until smooth.
3. Enjoy. Wow! You have ended the 9th day of your weight loss and detox journey.

Nutrition:

- 32 Calories
- 0.3g Fat
- 2g Protein
- 10mg Sodium
- 14g Carbohydrate
- Water
- 2g Fiber.

202. Kale Parsley and Chia Seeds Detox Smoothie

Preparation Time: 15 minutes
Cooking Time: 0
Servings: 1
Ingredients:

- Three tbsp. chia seeds (grounded)
- One cupful of water
- One sliced banana
- One pear (chopped)
- One cupful of organic kale
- One cupful of parsley
- Two tbsp. of lemon juice
- A dash of cinnamon

Directions:

1. Add the whole recipes together into a blender and pour the water before blending. Blend at high speed until smooth and enjoy. You may or may not place it in the refrigerator, depending on how hot or cold the weather appears.

Nutrition:

- 75 Calories
- 1g Fat
- 5g Protein
- 10g Fiber

Conclusion

Thank you for making it to the end of Dr. Sebi's book of recipes. Dr. Sebi's eating regimen is an antacid dinner plan, which is generally a veggie lover diet. The eating regimen depends on plants that control human-made weight control plans and cross breed nourishments as well. The eating regimen likewise guarantees that there are least degrees of corrosive in the nourishments you devour and the bodily fluid in one's body.

He additionally accepts that when individuals follow the two strategies, they make a domain, basic, not perfect for the endurance of maladies in the human body.

What inspired the specialist to receive the eating regimen is his starting point back in Honduras. The inspiration driving Dr. Sebi's eating routine focuses back to Alfredo Darrington Bowman (Dr. Sebi). He is a local Honduran, known as an intracellular specialist, botanist, and common healer.

Eating food is an everyday schedule that people should experience. The idea of substances and nourishments that we devour ordinary can bring about a lifetime utilization propensity on the off chance that it isn't directed. Before hopping into the basic way of life, you have to contemplate it. It will assist you with abstaining from making void vows to self.

This eating routine diminishes body contaminants and supports general prosperity. It will make you take a more secure, better way to deal with food.

It will likewise raise the odds of different infections. On the chance that you need to shed pounds, it can spur you to do it effectively and dependably. This is identified with improved quality and versatility that everybody requires.

Dr. Sebi's eating regimen is an altogether new way to deal with food. Thusly, it may be difficult to become acclimated to it, particularly toward the beginning.

It is prudent to attempt Dr. Sebi's Directions for 30 days if you don't completely receive another dietary system. Connect with for a month and see the upgrades. Following a month, you should change to this eating regimen altogether.

Dr. Sebi's diet advances eating entire, natural, plant-based food. Numerous people have used to cause a noteworthy change in their wellbeing. They are perfect in moving from acidic to soluble. You can similarly utilize them for occasionally keeping up your body framework and improving your wellbeing.

Not exclusively will you eat scrumptious suppers, you will likewise be helping yourself and your family to feel much improved and improve in general wellbeing just by eating affirmed Doctor Sebi's food. How incredible is that?

Now there is just one thing for you to do: Take action!

I hope you enjoyed reading this book. If you are looking to follow a more plant-based eating pattern, Dr. Sebi's diet has many healthy diets that are more flexible and sustainable.

I wish you great success in your journey for good health!

CPSIA information can be obtained
at www.ICGtesting.com
Printed in the USA
LVHW011652200221
679511LV00003B/325